OWNER'S MANUAL FOR THE HUMAN BODY
Revised Edition
Kundalini Yoga as Taught by Yogi Bhajan®

Compiled and Illustrated by: Harijot Kaur Khalsa

KRI Reviewer: Siri Neel Kaur Khalsa

Original Recordings: Siri Ved Singh Khalsa

Design & Production: Ravitej Singh Khalsa Design

Yogi Bhajan Photo: Satsimran Kaur

Published by **Kundalini Research Institute**, PO Box 1819, Santa Cruz, NM 87567
ISBN 978-1-934532-40-9

Acknowledgements

The technology of Kundalini Yoga was brought to the West from India by the grace of Yogi Bhajan. The teachings in this manual are entirely his gift to us. We wish to gratefully acknowledge his gift and inspiration to serve our highest human potential. Any errors or omissions in this manual are due to the editors and illustrator and do not reflect on the perfection and comprehensiveness of Yogi Bhajan's teachings.

The yoga sets in this manual are classes taught by Yogi Bhajan and recordings of most classes are available. Although every effort has been made to communicate the technology of these classes accurately in this manual, nothing replaces the experience of doing Kundalini Yoga with the Master, Yogi Bhajan.

We suggest that you enhance your yoga experience by collecting recordings of one or more of your favorite sets from this manual. There is something about doing Kundalini Yoga in the presence of the Master, Yogi Bhajan (even on recordings) that brings out the best yogi within you. See www.kundaliniresearchinstitute.org or www.a-healing.com for information about purchasing recordings of Yogi Bhajan's classes. Lectures and Yoga Classes with Yogi Bhajan are also available online at www.yogibhajan.org, the home of The Yogi Bhajan Library of Teachings.

We also wish to acknowledge the following people whose generous help brought about the original version of the Owner's Manual: Ardas Kaur Khalsa, Shakti Parwha Kaur Khalsa, Gurucharan Singh Khalsa, Pritpal Kaur Khalsa, Gobind Kaur Khalsa, Sada Sat Kaur Khalsa, and Kirpal Singh Khalsa.

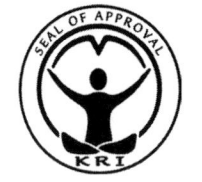

Introduction

For Beginners

If you are a beginning student of Kundalini Yoga as taught by Yogi Bhajan®, practicing for less than six months, or if you have been practicing without the aid of a KRI certified teacher, please read this introduction before you begin to practice from this instruction manual.

Sadhana Guidelines

This manual has been prepared as a supplement and extension to Kundalini Yoga Sadhana Guidelines, 2nd Edition, in which Yogi Bhajan explains yoga, meditation, and the energy that is Kundalini. Also important for beginners are the descriptions of the basics of Kundalini Yoga: asanas (postures), mudras (hand positions), bandhas (energy locks), and mantras (sound currents) written by Gurucharan Singh Khalsa, Director of Training for the Kundalini Research Institute's Aquarian Trainer Academy.

The Teacher

Kundalini Yoga is a spiritual discipline which cannot be practiced without a teacher. However it is not necessary for the teacher to be physically present when you practice. To establish a creative link with the Master of Kundalini Yoga, Yogi Bhajan, you should be sure to tune in to his energy flow using the Adi Mantra, *Ong Namo Guru Dev Namo.*

Tuning In

Every Kundalini Yoga session begins with chanting the Adi Mantra: *Ong Namo Guru Dev Namo.* By chanting it in its proper form and consciousness, the student becomes open to the higher Self, the source of all guidance, and accesses the protective link between himself or herself and the divine teacher.

How to Recite the Adi Mantra

Sit in a comfortable cross-legged position with the spine straight. Place the palms of the hands together as if in prayer, with the fingers pointing straight up, and then press the joints of the thumbs into the center of the chest, at the sternum. Inhale deeply. Focus your concentration at the root of the nose between the eyebrows, your Brow Point. As you exhale, chant the entire mantra in one breath. If your breath is not capable of this, take a quick sip of air through the mouth after "Ong Namo" and then chant the rest of the mantra, extending the sound as long as possible. The sound "Dev" is chanted a minor third higher than the other sounds of the mantra.

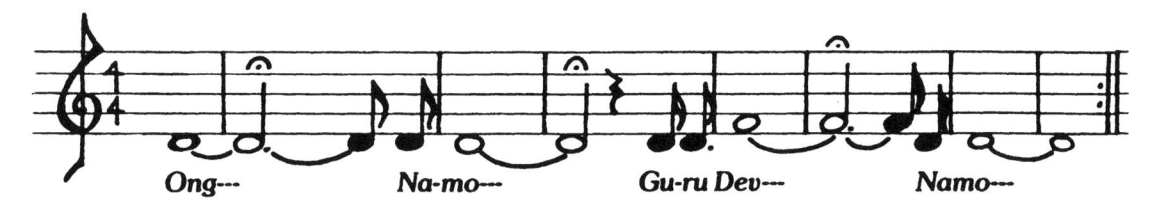

Ong---   Na-mo---   Gu-ru Dev---   Namo---

As you chant, vibrate the cranium with the sound to create a mild pressure at the Brow Point or third eye. Chant this mantra at least three times before beginning your Kundalini Yoga practice. See www.kriteachings.org to hear a sample of the Director of Training leading the Adi Mantra.

Pronunciation

The "O" sound in *Ong* is long, as in "go" and of short duration. The "ng" sound is long and produces a definite vibration on the roof of the mouth and cranium. The first part of *Namo,* is short and rhymes with "hum." The "O", as in "go" is held longer.
The first syllable of *Guru* is pronounced as in the word, "good." The second syllable rhymes with "true." The first syllable is short and the second one long. The word, *Dev,* rhymes with "gave."

Definition

Ong is the infinite creative energy experienced in manifestation and activity. It is a variation of the cosmic syllable *Om* which denotes God in an absolute or unmanifested state. God as Creator is called *Ong.*

Namo has the same root as the Sanskrit word *Namaste* which means reverent greetings.

Namaste is a common greeting in India accompanied by the palms pressed together at the chest or forehead. It implies bowing down. Together *Ong Namo* means "I call on the infinite creative consciousness," and opens you to the universal consciousness that guides all action.

Guru is the embodiment of the wisdom that one is seeking. The Guru is the giver of the technology. *Dev* means higher, subtle, or divine. It refers to the transparent or spiritual realms.

Namo, in closing the mantra, reaffirms the humble reverence of the student. Taken together, *Guru Dev Namo* means "I call on the divine wisdom," whereby you bow before your higher Self to guide you in using the knowledge and energy given by the cosmic Self.

Mental Focus

The following pages contain many wonderful techniques. To fully appreciate and receive the benefits of each one you will need mental focus. Unless you are directed to do otherwise, focus your concentration on the Brow Point, which is located between the eyebrows just above the root of the nose. With your eyes closed, mentally locate this point by turning your eyes gently upwards and inwards. Remain aware of your breath, your body posture, your movements, and any mantra you may be using, even as you center your awareness at the Brow Point or third eye.

Linking the Breath With a Mantra

A mantra is a sequence of sounds designed to direct the mind by their rhythmic repetition. To fully utilize the power of mantra, link the mantra with your breath cycle. A basic mantra is Sat Nam (rhymes with "But Mom"). *Sat Nam* means "Truth is my identity." Mentally repeat "Sat" as you inhale, and "Nam" as you exhale. In this way you filter your thoughts so that each thought has a positive resolution. Mantra makes it easier to keep up during strenuous exercises and adds depth to the performance of even the simplest ones.

Pacing Yourself

Kundalini Yoga often involves the rhythmic movement between two or more postures. Begin slowly, keeping a steady rhythm. Increase gradually, being careful not to strain. Usually the more you practice an exercise, the faster you can go. Just be sure that the spine has become warm and flexible before attempting rapid movements. It is important to be aware of your body and to be responsible for its well-being.

Concluding an Exercise

Unless otherwise stated, an exercise is concluded by inhaling and holding the breath briefly, then exhaling and relaxing the posture. While the breath is being held, apply the Mulbandh or Root Lock, contracting the muscles around the anus, the sex organs, and the Navel Point. This consolidates the effects of any exercise and circulates the energy to your higher centers. Do not hold the breath to the point of dizziness. If you start to feel dizzy or faint, immediately exhale and relax.

Relaxation Between Exercises

Yogi Bhajan taught many of the Kriyas in this manual with no breaks between the exercises. As in all Kriyas in Kundalini Yoga as taught by Yogi Bhajan®, rests may be taken in between exercises when appropriate unless the Kriya specifically states otherwise. Unless otherwise specified you should allow 1 to 3 minutes of relaxation in Easy Pose or lying on the back in Corpse Pose after each exercise. The less experienced you are or the more strenuous the exercise, the longer the relaxation period should be. Some sets end with a period of "deep relaxation" which may extend from 3 to 11 minutes.

Music and Mantras

See page 49 for information on where to get the music played in various sets. If you do not have the specific version played in a set you may substitute other meditative Kundalini Yoga music or do the set without music.

To hear the correct pronunciation of an individual mantra used in this manual, please visit www.kundaliniresearchinstitute.org and click on "Tools for Students and Teachers" and then on "Aquarian Teacher Mantra Pronunciation."

On Your Way...

The exercises in this manual are designed to be safe for most people, provided the instructions are followed carefully. The benefits attributed to these exercises come from centuries-old yogic tradition. Results will vary due to physical differences and the correctness and frequency of practice. The publishers and authors disclaim all liability in connection with the use of the information in individual cases. As with all unsupervised exercise programs, your use of the instructions in this manual is taken at your own risk. If you have any doubts as to the suitability of the exercises, please consult your doctor.

We invite you to now enjoy the practice of the Kundalini Yoga techniques contained in the following pages. If you have any questions or concerns about your practice of Kundalini Yoga, please contact your local KRI Certified Kundalini Yoga Teacher (online at www.kundaliniyoga.com)

VIII

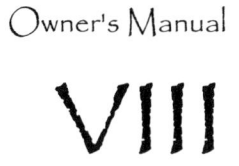

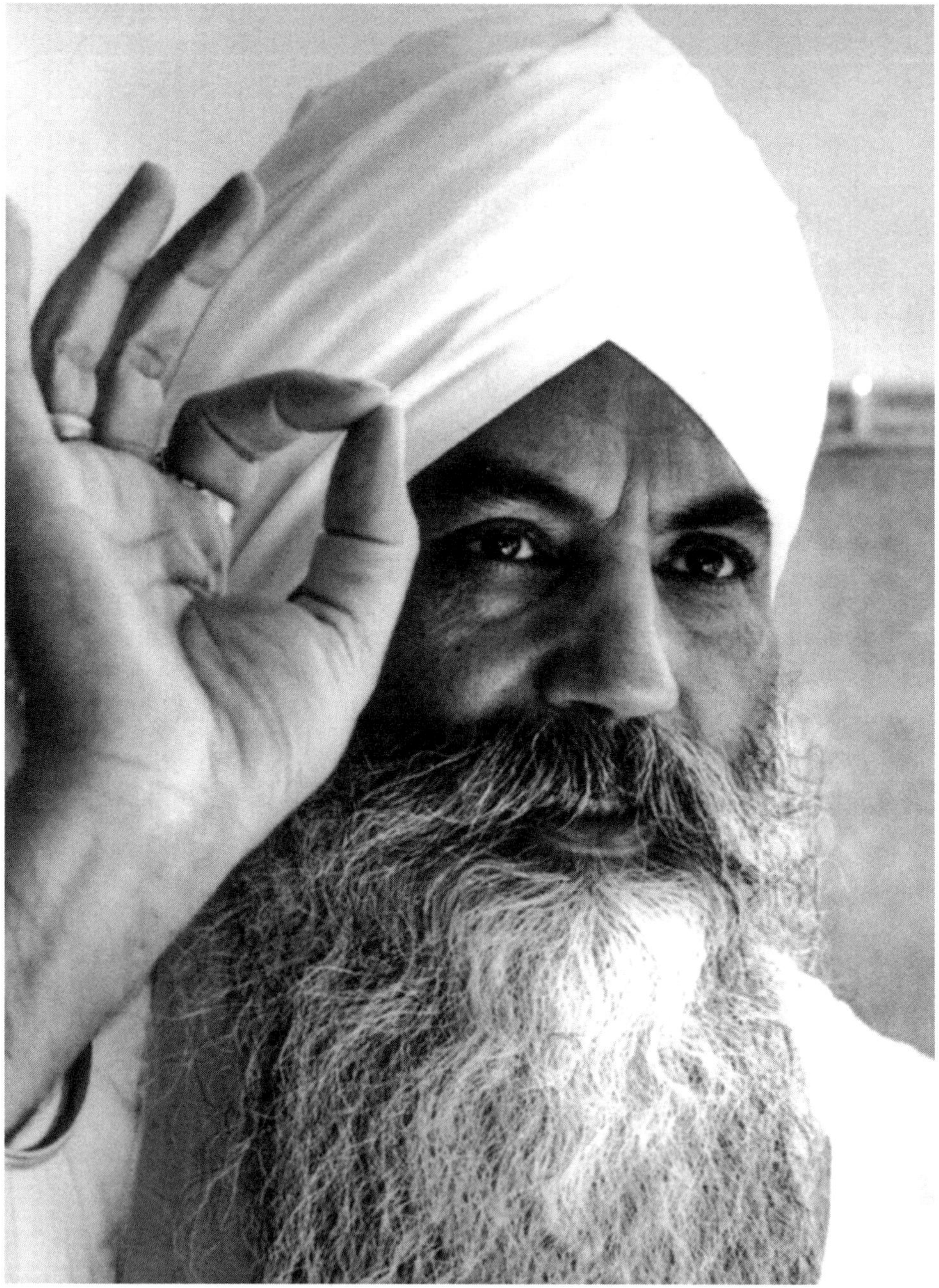

"Body is a good thing.
Use it until it obeys you."

Yogi Bhajan

Table of Contents

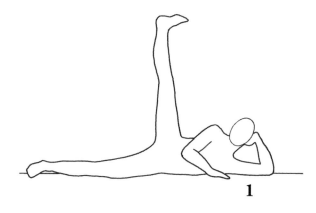

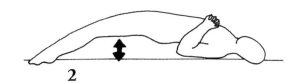

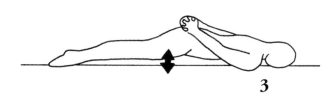

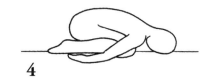

Automatic Endurance in the Body

October 12, 1988

Meditation: Conscious breath for total self-purification:

Sit in an easy meditative posture. Inhale through the nose for 20 seconds, hold the breath for 20 seconds, and exhale through the nose for 20 seconds. Start with 6 Minutes and gradually build the time up to 31 Minutes. "If you can do it for thirty-one minutes a day, and you can perfect it, in forty days or ninety days, you don't need anything else on this planet Earth... Period. It does it all."

Yoga Set:

1. Lie on your left side and raise the right leg all the way up. Keep both legs straight. Rest your head on your left hand. There will be pressure on your left elbow. Hold the position and inhale in eight strokes and exhale in eight strokes. The breath in this posture gives tolerance and grit. 3 Minutes.

2. Lie down flat on your back, lock your hands across your chest on top of your heart and jump the whole body up off the ground, while keeping the hands locked in place. Keep your legs straight. "Give your nervous system a shock treatment."
2 1/2 Minutes. Now, staying in the same posture, jump your body to the right, to the left, and up in three equal proportions and three dimensions. Hands have to be kept tightly locked. "Go mad...get all of the anger and tension out of your system. Develop nerves of steel."
2 1/2 Minutes.

3. Lie down on your belly and join your hands across your back and jump your whole body up off the floor. 2 1/2 Minutes.

4. Lie down in Baby Pose and sleep for 15 Minutes. (Yogi Bhajan played the gong for the last two minutes of this lay out.)

To Finish: Cat Stretch left and right. 30 Seconds.

"You can do this set every day, every morning. You will become, by right of your own doing and recognizing, divine human beings. There are two ways to live, folks. Live as divided persons or live as divine person. There is no alternative."

"You should, as a matter of rule, remain fifteen minutes minimum in Baby Pose if you want to live healthy. These are the requirements of a person: one apple a day, one banana a day, one orange a day, and fifteen minutes of Baby Pose."

The capacity of a human being is how much automatic endurance is in the body. The gift of God is that the body has to be carried every day with x amount of energy and sometimes it is not there. Sometimes the chips are down and sometime the chips are up. People do not understand that they have to stimulate themselves and their glandular system to add to the mix... (In ancient times) body was considered the Temple of God. Health was considered the gift of God. Man was considered the being of God.

Yogi Bhajan

1

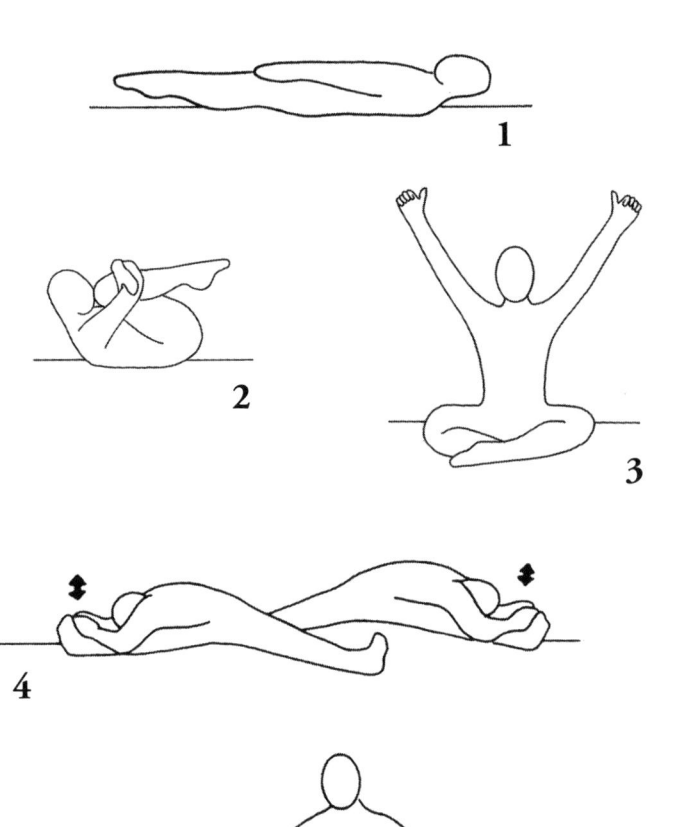

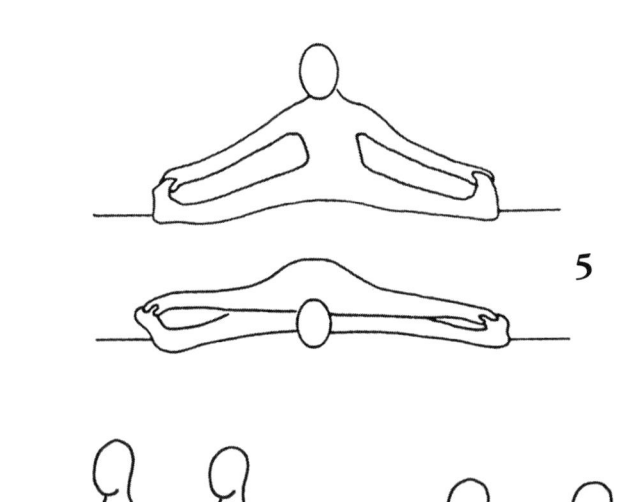

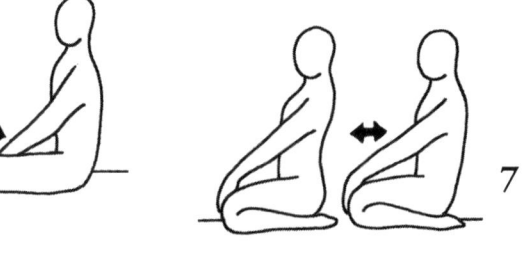

Awakening Yourself to Your Ten Bodies

2

1. Stretch Pose: lie on your back with your arms at your sides. Raise your head and your heels six inches and look at the tips of your toes. The hands are lifted with the palms held slightly above the hips facing each other. Point your toes and do Breath of Fire. 1-3 Minutes.

2. Hug your knees to your chest, with your arms wrapped around them. Tuck your nose between your knees, and begin Breath of Fire. 1-3 Minutes.

3. Sit in Easy Pose or in Celibate Pose. Raise your arms to a 60 degree angle and curl your fingers into the mounds at their base. Stretch your thumbs away from your palms. Keep your arms in a straight line from the shoulders through the wrists. Close your eyes, concentrate at the third eye point, and do Breath of Fire. 1-3 Minutes.

4. Sit with the legs stretched wide apart. Arms overhead, inhale, then exhale, stretch down and grab the toes of the left foot. Inhale and come straight up, and then exhale and stretch down over the right leg and grab the toes. Continue 1-3 Minutes.

5. Continue to sit with the legs stretched wide apart. Hold onto the toes, inhale and sit up straight. Exhale and stretch down bringing the chest toward the floor. Then inhale, rise up, and continue. 1-3 Minutes.

6. Spinal Flex in Easy Pose: grab your shins in front with both hands. Inhale. Extend the spine forward, rocking forward on your buttocks. Then exhale, flex the spine backwards and roll back on your buttocks. Keep your head level and your arms fairly straight but relaxed. 1-3 Minutes.

7. Spinal Flex sitting on your heels: place your hands flat on your thighs. Flex the spine forward on the inhale, backward on the exhale. Focus at the third eye point. 1-3 Minutes.

The Ten Bodies:
Soul Body
Negative Mind
Positive Mind
Neutral Mind
Physical Body
Arc Line
Auric Body
Pranic Body
Subtle Body
Radiant Body

Yogi Bhajan

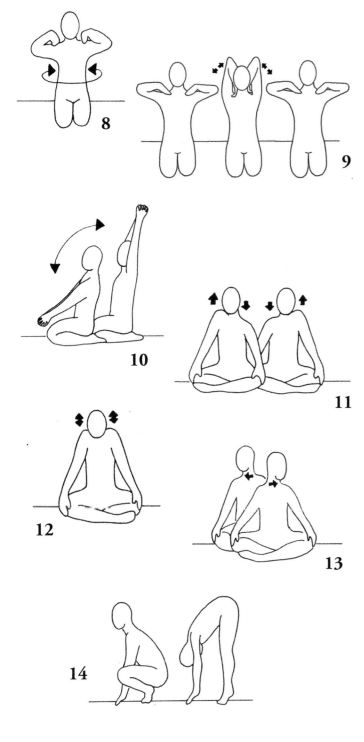

8. Spinal twist sitting on your heels: grasp your shoulders with the fingers in front, thumbs in back. Inhale and twist to the left, exhale and twist to the right. Keep your upper arms parallel to the floor. 1-3 Minutes.

9. Grasp the shoulders as in the previous exercise. Inhale and raise the elbows up so that the backs of the wrists touch behind the neck. Exhale and lower the elbows to the original position. 1-3 Minutes.

10. Interlace the fingers in Venus Lock. Inhale and stretch the arms up over the head, then exhale and bring the hands back toward the lap, but do not touch it. 1-3 Minutes.

11. Sit in Easy Pose with your hands resting on your knees. Inhale and shrug the left shoulder up, then exhale and raise the right shoulder up as you lower the left shoulder. Continue for 1 Minute. Then, reverse the breath so that you inhale as you shrug the right shoulder up, exhale as you shrug the left shoulder up and lower the right shoulder. Continue for 1 Minute.

12. Inhale and shrug both shoulders up, exhale while relaxing them down. 1 Minute

13. Remain sitting in Easy Pose with your hands on your knees. Inhale, and twist your head to the left, and exhale and twist it to the right, like shaking your head "no". Continue for 1 Minute. Then reverse your breath, so that you inhale and twist to the right, and exhale and twist to the left. Continue for 1 Minute. Inhale deeply, concentrate at the third eye, and slowly exhale.

14. Frog Pose: squat down so your buttocks are on your heels. Your heels are off the ground and touching each other. Put your fingertips on the ground between your knees. Keep your head up. Inhale, straighten your legs, keeping the fingers on the ground. Exhale and come back into a squat facing forward. The inhale and exhale should be strong. Do 54 Frogs.

15. Deeply relax on the back.

Laya Yoga Meditation

Sit in Easy Pose with your hands on your knees in Gyan Mudra (thumb and index finger touching.) Chant the mantra: Ek Ong Kar-ah, Sa Ta Na Ma-ah, Siri Wha-ah Hay Guru. The "ah" sound is created by pulling Mul Bhand (pulling in on the navel while simultaneously pulling up on the rectum and sex organs). When the navel is strongly drawn in as you are chanting, it produces an exhalation which sounds like "ah". As you chant, visualize the sound spiraling up the spine from the base to the top of the head in 3 1/2 circles. 11-31 Minutes.

Balancing the Vayus

February 12, 1986

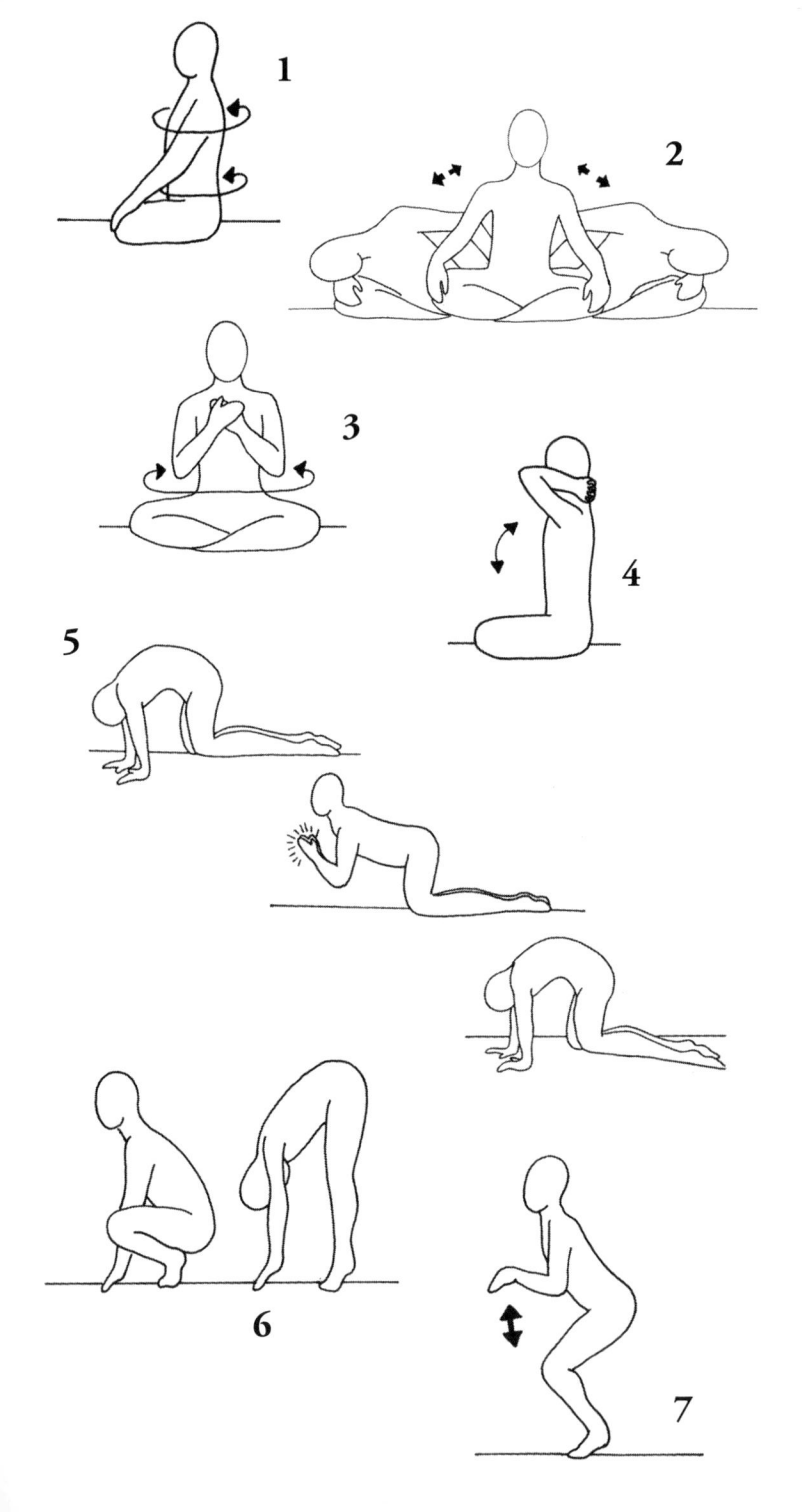

There are five principal Vayus: Praana, which moves in the heart area, Udaana in the throat; Samaana in the navel region; Apaana in the pelvic floor area; and Vyaana which circulates throughout the whole body. These five Vayus have to have a combination and a balance. This set moves all the Vayus of the body and brings an equilibrium to the entire glandular system.

"If you can just practice this one set alone, you will be surprised how much control on your mind, body and soul, and how much combination you can achieve."

1. Sit in Easy Pose. Put your hands on your knees, keeping your spine straight and stretched upward. Keep your arms straight. Create a small circular motion at the base of your spine. The circular movement of the upper body is not broader than that at the base of the spine. Don't let the spine bend, so that the movement of the whole spine is governed by the circling movement at your base.

2. Stay in Easy Pose with your hands on your knees. Bend to the left, touching your forehead to your left knee. Rise up and then bend to the right, touching your forehead to your right knee. Rise up and continue 1 Minute.

3. Stay in Easy Pose and place both hands, one on top of the other, at your heart center touching your chest. Twist your body left and right, moving from your navel point, using your shoulders as a fulcrum. 1 Minute.

4. Still in Easy Pose, lock your hands behind your neck, keep your spine straight, and bend forward toward the ground and rise up. Move quickly and rhythmically. 1 Minute.

5. Get into Cat-Cow position and begin flexing your spine up and down as rapidly as you can for 15 Seconds. Then, as your head comes up in Cow, lift your hands from the ground and clap. As your head bows down in Cat, return your hands to the ground. Continue 1 Minute.

6. Squat down in Frog Pose with your heels together and your fingertips on the floor between your knees. Balance on the balls of your feet. Inhale and straighten your legs, exhale and return to the squatting position. Do 21 Frogs.

7. Stand like a kangaroo with your knees bent and your arms close to the sides bent at the elbows and wrists so that your arms look like a kangaroo's forepaws. From this position, jump up and down. Do 21 Kangaroo Jumps.

There are two ways to go in your life: one is to 'go and get it' and the other one is to 'be and get it.' One is to develop your physical body to go for everything. Other is to develop your radiant body so that everything will come to you. And the best way is to develop (both) your radiant body and your physical body so that you can have perfect balance.

Yogi Bhajan

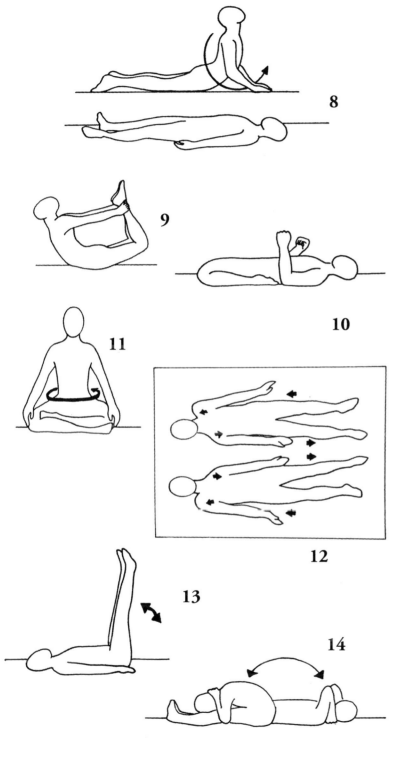

8. Lie on your stomach with your heels together and your hands on the ground under your shoulders. Rise up into Cobra Pose. From Cobra Pose quickly roll your body to the left so that you end up lying on your back on the ground. Roll back onto your stomach and rise back up into Cobra Pose. This time roll your body to the right, rolling quickly over so that you again end up on your back on the ground. Roll back onto your stomach, up into Cobra Pose, and continue. 1 1/2 Minutes.

9. Lie on your stomach and grab your ankles. Press your legs away and raise your chest up, coming up into Bow Pose. Begin a strong Breath of Fire so that your belly button moves. 1 Minute.

10. Sit on your heels, and then spread your knees, placing your buttocks on the ground between the heels. Lie back so that your upper body is on the ground. With your fists begin drumming your upper chest (the lymph area) for 20 Seconds, then gently drum on your belly for 15 Seconds, then heavily drum your thighs for 15 Seconds, then gently drum your navel point for 10 Seconds, and then drum both sides of your neck for 15 Seconds.

11. Sit once more in Easy Pose with your hands on your knees. Rotate your upper body 51 times counter-clockwise, squeezing the digestive area.

12. Lie down flat on your back. Extend your left hip and shoulder downward while you stretch your right hip and shoulder upward. Then extend your right hip and shoulder downward toward your feet while stretching your left hip and shoulder upward. Move diagonally and move powerfully. 2 Minutes.

13. Still lying on your back bring your knees straight and your heels together. Lift your legs up to 90 degrees and lower them back down with Breath of Fire. Move quickly. 1 1/4 Minutes.

14. Still on your back, lock your hands behind your neck and rise up straight. Bend forward, bringing your upper body down to your thighs and then lie back down flat. Move quickly and continue this movement for 1 1/2 Minutes.

15. Lie down flat and completely relax your body for 11 Minutes. "Feel the shakti (energy) moving in your spine... from your tailbone to the top of your head." Listen to Bhai Avatar Singh's version of "Je Teh Gung." Yogi Bhajan played the gong to further activate the shakti energy.

Complete Workout For the Total Self

March 21, 1984

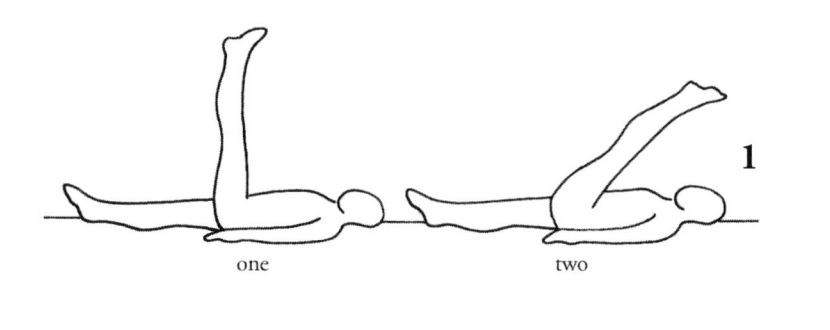

one   two   1

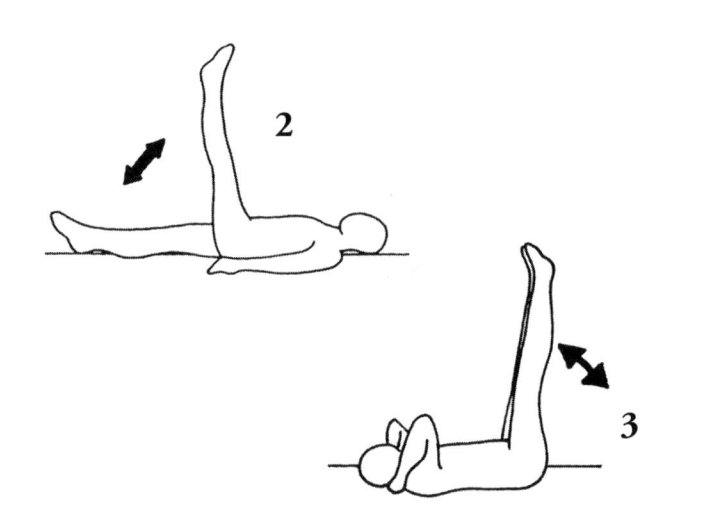

2

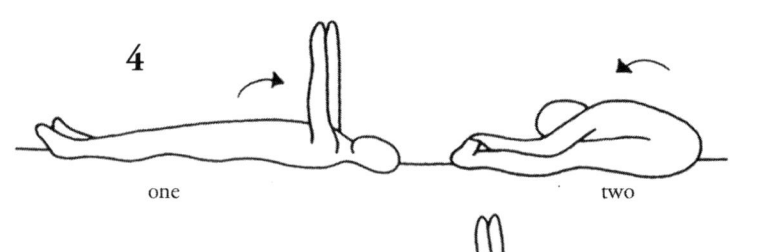

3

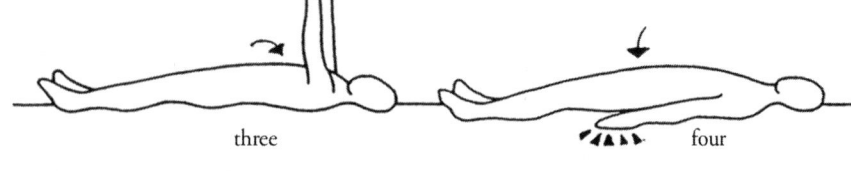

4   one   two

three   four

1. Lie down on the back with arms relaxed at the sides, palms down. Raise the left leg straight up to a 90 degree angle, allowing the rest of the body to be relaxed. Keeping the leg straight and without using your hands, bring your leg towards your head on the count of "one" and on the count of "two" bring it back to ninety degrees. Continue counting and moving in this manner from one to eight and then start counting back from eight to one. (8-count = 4 seconds) Continue in this way, counting aloud, for 1 1/2 Minutes. Without breaking rhythm, change sides and repeat the exercise with the right leg for 1 1/2 Minutes. (This repeat was added later by Yogi Bhajan so this exercise may be done either only with left leg as taught in class or with both the left and right legs as taught later.)

2. Remaining on your back, lift the left leg up to 90 degrees, keeping the knee straight, on the count of "one". On the count of "two", touch the left heel to the ground, on "three" raise the left leg up again and on "four" lower it back to the ground. Continue in this way, raising and lowering the left leg only, using an 8-count out loud. (8-count = 6 seconds) After 2 1/2 Minutes change sides, without breaking the rhythm, and raise and lower the right leg in the same manner for 1 Minute.

3. Remaining on the back, interlock your hands behind your neck and bring both legs together with the knees straight and the heels together. On the count of "one" raise both legs up to 90 degrees and on the count of "two" return them to the ground. Continue, raising and lowering the legs using a quick 8-count out loud for 3 Minutes.

4. Be on your back with your arms at the sides: On the count of "one", raise both arms up to 90 degrees, parallel to each other, palms facing foward. On "two", sit up and touch your fingers to your toes (knees straight). On "three", return to position on your back with your arms up at 90 degrees, and on "four", bring your arms down to hit the ground along side your body. (4-count = 6 seconds) Continue, keeping rhythm as you count aloud. 4 Minutes.

Yoga is a science and it is not 'exercises.' What a yoga exercise can do is move your muscle to muscle, nerve to nerve, meridian point to meridian point. Actually it is to stimulate the glands in the proper areas so that there is no confusion in health.

Yogi Bhajan

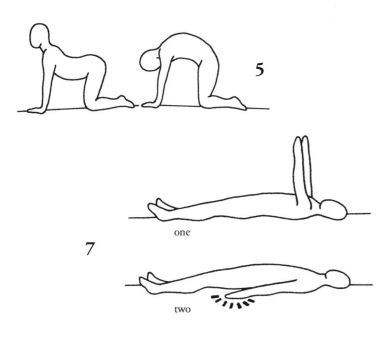

5. Be on the hands and knees, with heels touching. Inhale and arch the spine down into Cow Pose so that the head comes way up, and on the exhale arch up into Cat Pose so that the chin comes into the chest. Breathe very powerfully, keeping rhythm to mental count (or leader may count aloud) of 1 through 8. (8-count = 4-6 seconds) 2 Minutes.

6. Relax on the back for 1 Minute. Create the feeling that you are peaceful and very grateful.

7. Stay on your back. On the count of "one" raise your arms up to 90 degrees, with the palms facing forward. On "two", bring your arms down to the sides, so that the palms slap the ground with enough force to make a noise.(2-count = 2 seconds) Keep the rest of your body relaxed. 1 1/2 Minutes. Then continue the action adding the Snake Breath (inhale deeply through the nostrils, and exhale making a hissing sound by forcing the breath through the teeth, with the tongue pressing lightly against the back of the teeth. The lips will pull back slightly to let the air escape.) for 1 1/2 Minutes more, keeping the arms and breath going in rhythm.

8. Sit up in Easy Pose with your spine straight. Place your hands on your shoulders with the fingers are in front and thumbs in back, elbows and upper arms parallel to the ground. Inhale and twist to the left. Exhale and twist to the right. Keep the elbows up and breathe powerfully, moving the lymph gland area. 4 Minutes.

9. Sit in Celibate Pose, with the buttocks on the floor between the heels. Lock your hands behind your neck. On the count of "one" exhale and bring the forehead to the floor. On "two" inhale and rise back up. (2-count = 2 seconds) 2 Minutes.

10. Lie on your stomach, legs straight and heels together. On the count of "one," place your hands under your shoulders and push up into Cobra Pose, straightening the arms, arching the spine back. On "two," quickly come down flat with the chin touching the floor. On the count of "one" come back up into Cobra Pose. (2-count = 2-3 seconds) Use the Snake Breath, "the sound must come out of you like a big Cobra snake." Breathe powerfully and move with control. 4 Minutes.

11. Lie flat on your stomach and relax. Be in peace. 1 Minute.

Continued next page.

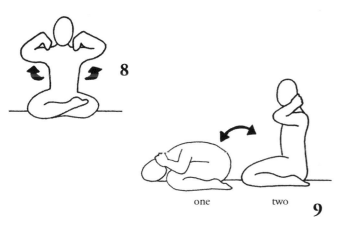

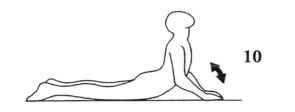

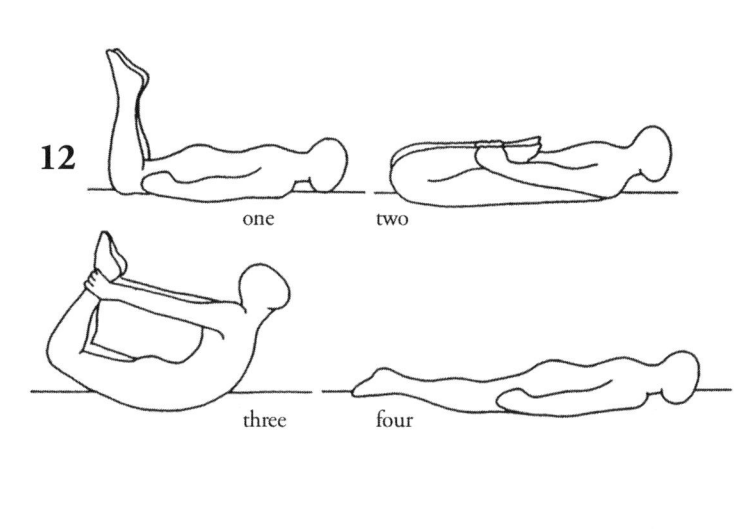

12

one   two

three   four

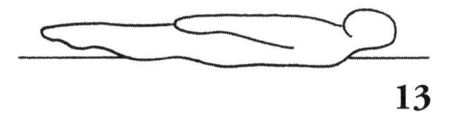

13

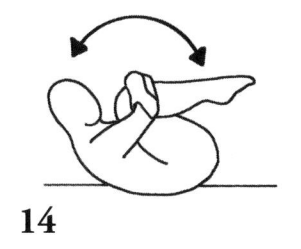

14

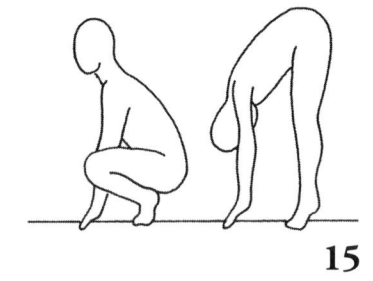

15

12. Stay on your stomach. On the count of "one" bend your knees and raise your feet up in the air. On "two", grab your ankles with your hands. On "three" arch up into Bow Pose, spreading the arch along your entire spine. On "four", release everything and lie flat on your stomach. (4-count = 4-6 seconds) Count out loud. 3 1/2 Minutes.

13. Come flat onto your back, heels together, arms at your sides. Come into Stretch Pose with your head and heels 6 inches from the floor, fingers pointing towards your toes. Begin a very powerful Breath of Fire. Let the navel area shake. 1 Minute.

14. Lying on your back, pull your knees into your chest, locking them in place with your hands. Begin Spinal Rolls, fully rolling back and forth on your spine. On the count of "one" roll up to sitting without releasing the posture and on the count of "two" roll back down the spine without releasing the arms. (2 count = 2 seconds) 2 Minutes.

15. Start in Frog Pose, squatting on the balls of your feet with your heels touching and your knees spread wide apart. Your arms come straight down between your knees, your fingertips rest on the floor and your head is up. On the count of "one," raise your buttocks, keeping the fingertips on the floor, and the knees straight. (Your head will be down.) On "two," return to squatting. Continue, keeping rhythm quickly counting from one to eight out loud with the movement. (8-count = 8 seconds) 1 1/2 Minutes.

16. Sit in Easy Pose. Close your eyes and vibrate the sound "Har Har, Har Har, Har Ha-Ray" in a monotone. (one complete mantra = 2-3 seconds) Power the vibration by using the navel point. 4 Minutes.

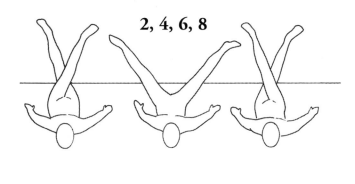

2, 4, 6, 8

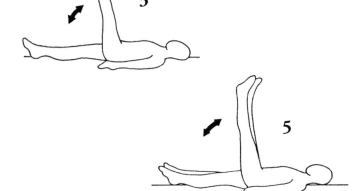

3

5

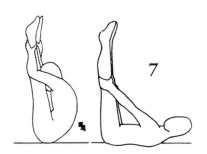

7

Nervous System Overhaul

December 5, 1985

1. Lie on your back and breathe very long, deeply and slowly. 1 Minute.

2. Still lying on your back raise your legs up to 90 degrees and criss-cross them rapidly with Breath of Fire. Breathe powerfully and move at the rate of the breath. 1 1/2 Minutes.

3. Begin alternate leg lifts to 90 degrees rapidly with Breath of Fire. Move your legs with the rate of your breath. Keep your legs straight. 3 Minutes.

4. Repeat exercise #2, criss-crossing your legs rapidly with Breath of Fire. Move quickly. 30 Seconds.

5. Now raise both legs together up to 90 degrees and lower them rapidly with Breath of Fire. Move your legs and your breath at the same time. 3 Minutes. This is very good for the nervous system.

6. Repeat exercise #2, criss-crossing your legs rapidly with Breath of Fire. Move quickly. 30 Seconds.

7. Raise your legs up to 90 degrees, balance on your buttocks, grab your calves with your hands and bring your nose to your knees. Exhale and lower your torso and then inhale and bring your nose back to your knees. Breath of Fire. 2 1/2 Minutes. This exercise "seals the energy in every organ of the body and recreates the lymph area."

8. Lie back with your legs still up at 90 degrees and criss-cross your legs briefly (10 seconds). Then lower your legs and relax. Yogi Bhajan played the gong during this meditation. 4 1/2 minutes. Then inhale and do some Cat Stretches left and right before getting up.

Breathing in this set is very powerful. "They call it 'agni yam', actually. They don't even call it 'agni praanayam.' They call it 'agni yam.' You create that much heat and fire that you can burn out anything which is anti-body in the fifteen minutes (that it takes to do this set)."

This one set can make you the best living person on the planet. All of the nervous system will be shaped up and balanced up. No breakdown.

Yogi Bhajan

Energize Your System

January 5, 1988

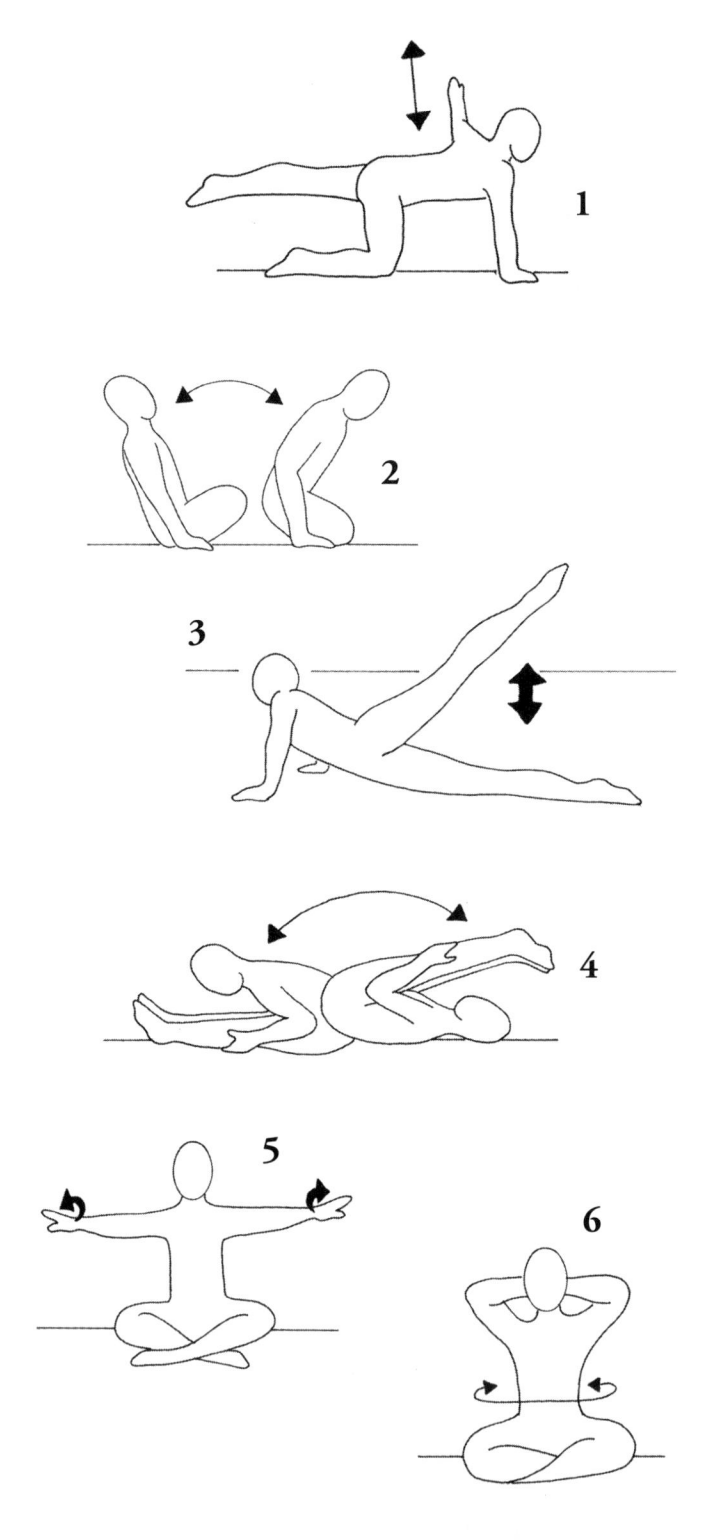

1. Kneel on your hands and knees. Raise your left arm up and out to the side. Raise your left leg straight out behind you parallel to the ground. (Take 30 seconds or so to stabilize yourself in the posture.) Hold the position and begin moving the left arm up and down very hard and fast. Your range of movement should be three feet. After a while your breath will automatically become a powerful Breath of Fire. Breathe from the navel. 2 1/2 Minutes. Change sides, lifting the right arm and leg and continue the rapid arm movement for 1 Minute. Change sides again, returning to the original position and continue 30 Seconds.

This movement energizes the heart chakra and the stomach, gives power to the immune system, and stimulates the thyroid and parathyroid.

2. Come into Easy Pose and place your hands palm down on the floor beside your hips. Put your weight on your hands and bend backward and forward as far as you can. (Your body will lift off the floor.) Keep moving without lifting your hands from the floor. 2 1/2 Minutes. This movement adjusts the spine.

3. Come into Cobra Pose. Lift your left leg as high as possible, allowing the left hip to lift and twist. Lower the left leg and raise the right leg as high as possible and continue alternating sides for 3 Minutes. Keep your knees straight but allow the hips to lift and roll with the movement. This exercise cleanses the liver.

4. Sit down and stretch your legs out straight. With your palms up, grab your legs under the knees and press the hands hard. Without bending the knees, roll back onto your back, bringing your legs toward the floor behind your head. Then roll up and bend forward bringing your head to your knees. Continue this movement for 2 Minutes. This exercise purifies the blood and brings color to your cheeks.

5. Come into Easy Pose with the arms straight out to the sides parallel to the ground, palms down. Rotate your arms backward in small circles very rapidly, keeping the elbows straight. (Move so fast that your hands become a blur.)
2 1/2 Minutes.

6. Still sitting in Easy Pose, lock your hands behind your head and twist left and right from the base of your spine. 1 Minute. Move powerfully.

The idea was to teach Americans something which will be good for their generations. It takes a very short time to become a good adept in yoga. Yoga has been defined to you in many ways, but let me define it to you in a very simple language. When you can relate to your Consciousness and your Consciousness can deliver to all concerned that which is you, that is called the opening of the 3rd eye. And that gives you intuition, productivity, self-confidence, and compassion. Minus that, you shall fail. Doesn't matter what other tactics you use.

Yogi Bhajan

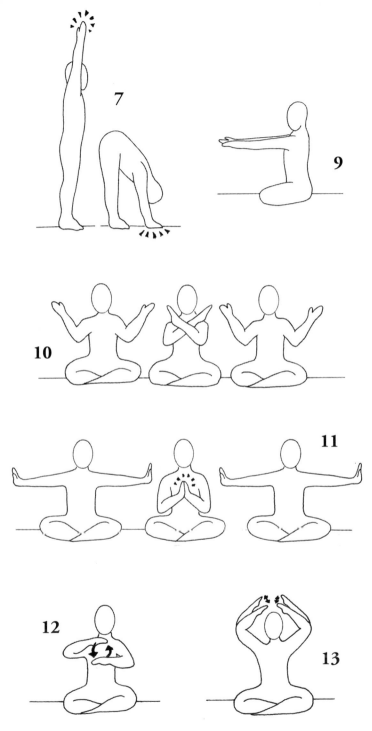

7. Stand up. Place your hands straight over your head and clap, then bend down quickly, keeping the knees straight, and hit the ground with your hands. Continue this movement 108 times. (One repetition = 1 second)

8. Lie down in Corpse Pose, cover up and relax for 22 Minutes. In the class, Yogi Bhajan played the gong and a variety of meditation songs. To wake up: roll your hands and feet and roll on your spine. (1 Minute)

9. Sit in Easy Pose and stretch both arms forward, parallel to the ground, with the left palm facing down and the right palm facing upward. Close your eyes and meditate to meditative music for 3 1/2 Minutes. This is to equalize the energy.

10. Allowing your arms to be comfortably bent at the elbows, begin criss-crossing your hands rapidly in front of your body. It's a clapping motion, but the hands don't touch. They pass by each other, alternating which hand passes on the outside. 1 1/2 Minutes. (This action symbolically means "let the sickness go.")

The meditative music continues playing.

11. Stretch your arms out to the sides, parallel to the ground, bend the wrists so that the palms are facing outward, fingertips pointing toward the ceiling. Bring the hands to the center of your chest and clap and return to the stretched position. Move quickly. 30 Seconds.

12. Begin revolving the hands around each other in an outward motion in front of your chest, moving fast enough to feel the wind on your face.(The meditative music continues playing.) 1 1/2 Minutes.

13. Raise your arms up to make an arc around your head. The elbows are bent and the hands are about 9" above your head. With both hands, begin patting the air above your head as if you were blessing yourself. The movement is small and subtle. 1 Minute. Inhale and tense the posture like steel, hold the breath for 30 Seconds. Exhale, inhale, tense the posture ("put all the energy into it"), and hold the breath 15 Seconds. Exhale, inhale, hold the breath, and make the posture "really tough" for 20 Seconds. Exhale and relax.

11

Working on the Lower Spine

April 24, 1985

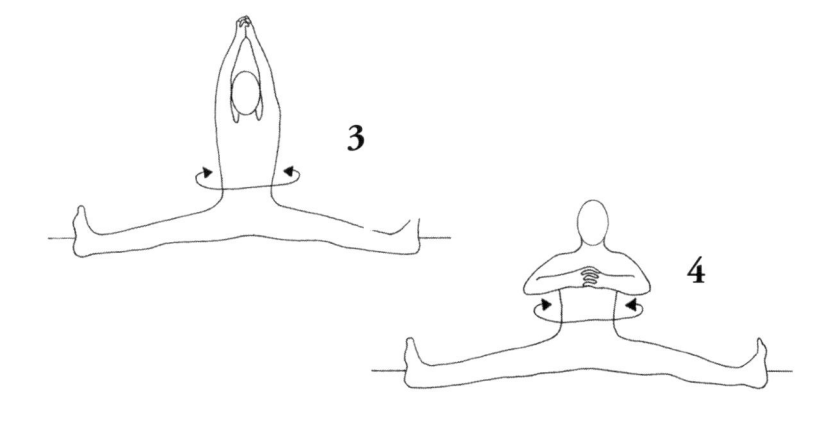

Haray

Har   Har

1

Haray   Har   Har

2

3

4

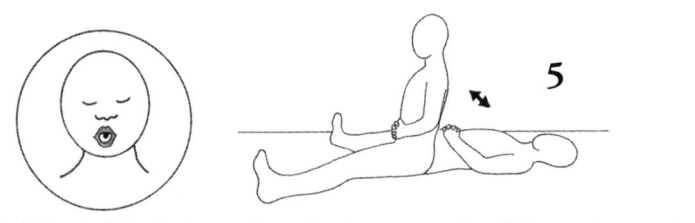

5

Sitali Style Breath of Fire: Pucker your lips and curl your tongue like a "U" protruding just a little beyong the lips. Breath through the tube-like opening made by the tongue and lips.

At the beginning of this class, Yogi Bhajan said that if anyone had a preexisting medical condition of the lower spine, they should not participate.

1. Sit on the floor and spread your legs as wide as possible. Interlock your hands behind your back. Bend to the left and touch the nose to the left knee and come up. Then bend to the right and touch the nose to the right knee and come up. As you bend over each knee the arms lift up. Move from your lower spine. Chant "Har" as you bend down and "Haray" as you come up. 4 1/2 Minutes. "This exercise is essential for your body... a basic elementary limbering exercise."

2. Without changing the posture, bend forward and chant "Har" as you touch your nose to your left knee and rise up. Bend down again to the center and chant "Har" and come up. Bend to the right knee and chant "Haray" and come up. Quick action! Continue for 1 1/2 Minutes.

3. Keeping your legs spread wide, raise the arms straight over the head and lock the hands. Twist the torso rapidly left and right keeping the arms straight. Rotate around your center line, moving the entire spine, not only the neck. "Go crazy, get mad!" This loosens up the lower rib cage and lungs. 2 1/2 Minutes.

4. Keeping the legs spread wide, lock your hands in front of your chest, palms facing down, and twist left and right. Use anger to fuel this movement. It is not a gentle movement, it has to be wild. Get your anger out. 2 Minutes.

5. Lie down on your back with the legs still spread wide, interlock your fingers, and rest both hands at your navel point. Hold your navel tight. Roll the tongue, stick it out of the mouth (as in Sitali Kriya) and do Breath of Fire through the mouth while raising and lowering your torso like a sit-up. Move up and down like a steam engine. Keep your legs straight. 5 Minutes. This exercise can keep your blood pressure balanced.

If your lower sciatica is tied down, it won't let your brain work. It won't let your day be good. It will mess up your nervous system. Your liver won't function right. Your circulatory organ will be totally uptight. Your lungs won't absorb the oxygen into the blood as they should... This is why those Hindus living on the Ganga's banks are beautiful. Because they do this (in the) early morning...They call on God, they meditate, and they stretch their thing, whatever the thing is. So at night they can sleep good.

Yogi Bhajan

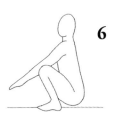

6

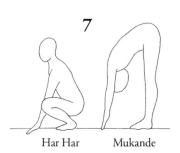

7

Har Har   Mukande

6. Come sitting in Crow Pose. Hold the position and concentrate on the third eye point. 2 1/2 Minutes. This posture was held during the affirmations section of the version of "Har Har Mukande (with affirmations)" by Liv Singh Khalsa that continues in the next exercise.

7. Stay in a squatting position with your hands on the ground. You are still meditating to "Har Har Mukande (with affirmations)" by Liv Singh Khalsa. Once the mantra starts, at each "Har Har" strongly pull in your navel point in the squatting position and at each "Mukande" straighten the knees and lift up the buttocks. 2 1/2 Minutes. This tunes all the organs of the body. (One "Har Har Mukande" = 3 seconds)

8. Relax 2 Minutes.

9. Sit and meditate at your third eye point for 1 1/2 Minutes. (Yogi Bhajan played the gong.)

This kriya is called "Apaana Chalunee Kriya." Yogi Bhajan said, "It is a very wonderful kriya. It is beautiful. It is written and sung and praised like anything...If it is properly done as it is and it is scaled, it is a must in a human life. It keeps the entire organ system of the body tuned up. After ten or fifteen days of doing it, I don't think you can be the same person as when you started. There is not one gland or one organ in the body that cannot be totally tuned up." By "scaled" Yogi Bhajan meant that the kriya can be expanded by proportionately extending the first four exercises to half an hour: #1 would be nine minutes; #2 would be three minutes; #3 & #4 would each be four minutes; and #5 would be ten minutes. Exercise #6 would be two minutes listening to the affirmations and twenty-eight minutes of Frogs with the navel pumping. This makes the total time for the kriya to be one hour.

Get Up and Get Going

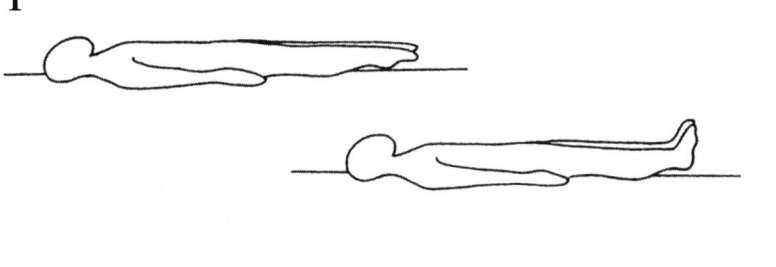

The exercise set can be done in your bed and will set you for the whole day.*

1. Lying on your back in bed, begin moving your feet in unison, flexing and pointing. 3 Minutes.

2. Lift both legs to approximately a 70 degree angle. Continue raising and lowering both legs for 3 Minutes.

3. Bring both legs up to 90 degrees, spread them as wide apart as you can. Keeping them spread apart, lower them to the bed. When they touch the bed, bring them together again. Continue for 3 Minutes.

4. Turn over and lie on your stomach with your arms by your sides and your head turned to one side. Begin kicking the buttocks with alternate heels. 3 Minutes.

5. Still on your stomach, begin raising and lowering the pelvic area, leaving the knees and shoulders touching the bed. This movement is done rapidly for 3 Minutes.

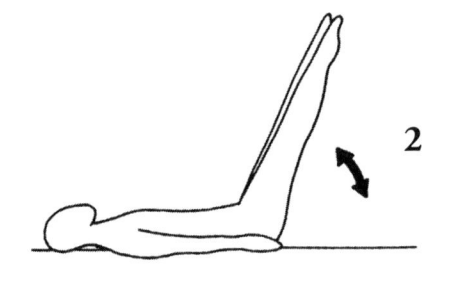

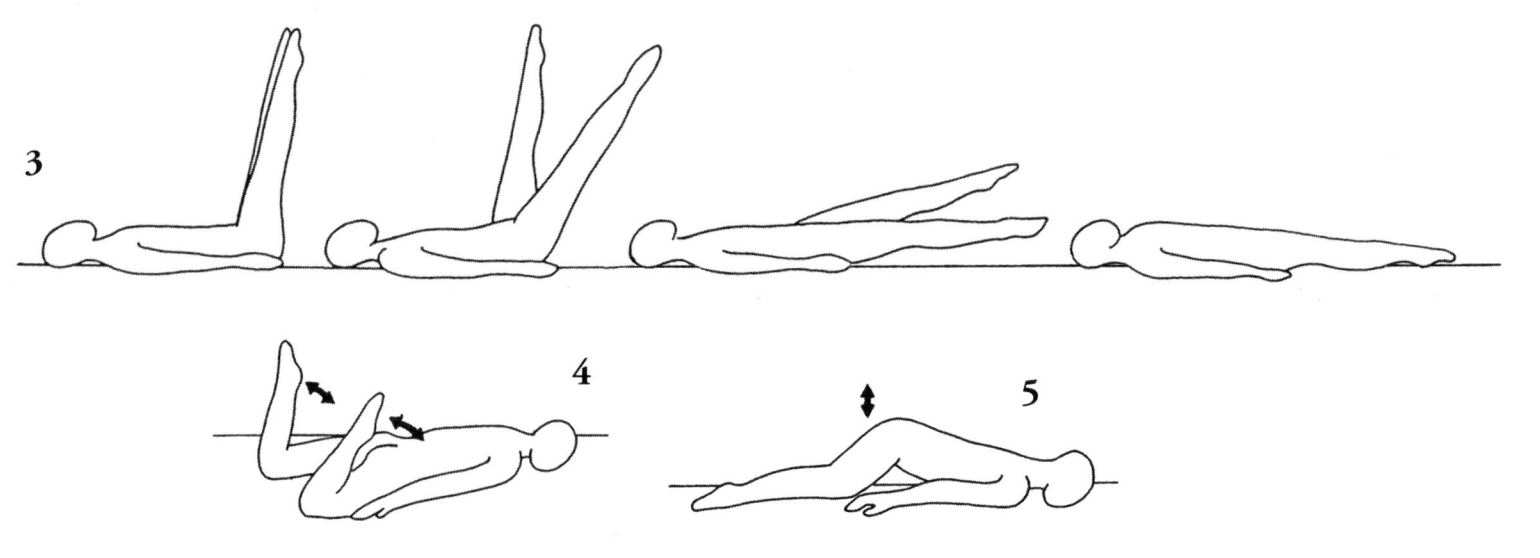

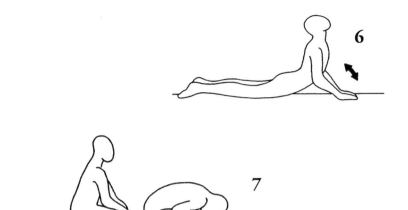

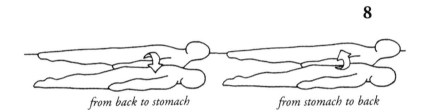

from back to stomach   *from stomach to back*

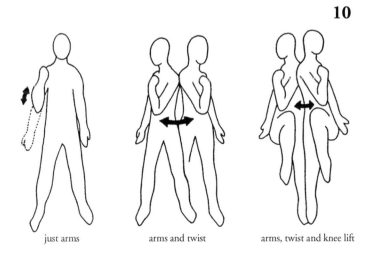

just arms   arms and twist   arms, twist and knee lift

6. With hands on either side of your chest, raise up into Cobra Pose. Do push-ups into a relaxed Cobra Pose for 3 Minutes.

7. Sit in Easy Pose with your hands on your knees. From the sitting position bring your forehead to the bed and then return to the upright position. 20 Times.

8. Do Bundle Roll: Lie on your back on your bed with your legs together and your arms at your sides as if you are a bundle of logs tied together. Flip yourself over from back to stomach and from stomach to back without bending the body, arms or legs. Do not bend anywhere. 3 Minutes.

9. Get out of bed.

10. Stand in front of a mirror. Have your arms at your sides with the palms of your hands facing forward. Make a fist of your right hand and bend your elbow, bringing your fist to your shoulder. Lower your right hand and relax the fist while you make a fist of your left hand and bring it to your shoulder. Continuing this movement, twist your torso from the waist: twisting to the left when your right fist comes up and twisting to the right when your left fist comes up. Once those two movements are coordinated, begin lifting the left knee up as you twist to the left and bring the right fist up. As you twist to the right, bring the right knee up as the left fist comes up. This is to be aerobic movement so move quickly. 3 Minutes.

11. Take your shower and begin your day.

* The instructions for this kriya are from the contemporaneous notes of Satsimran Kaur and could not be verified by KRI review.

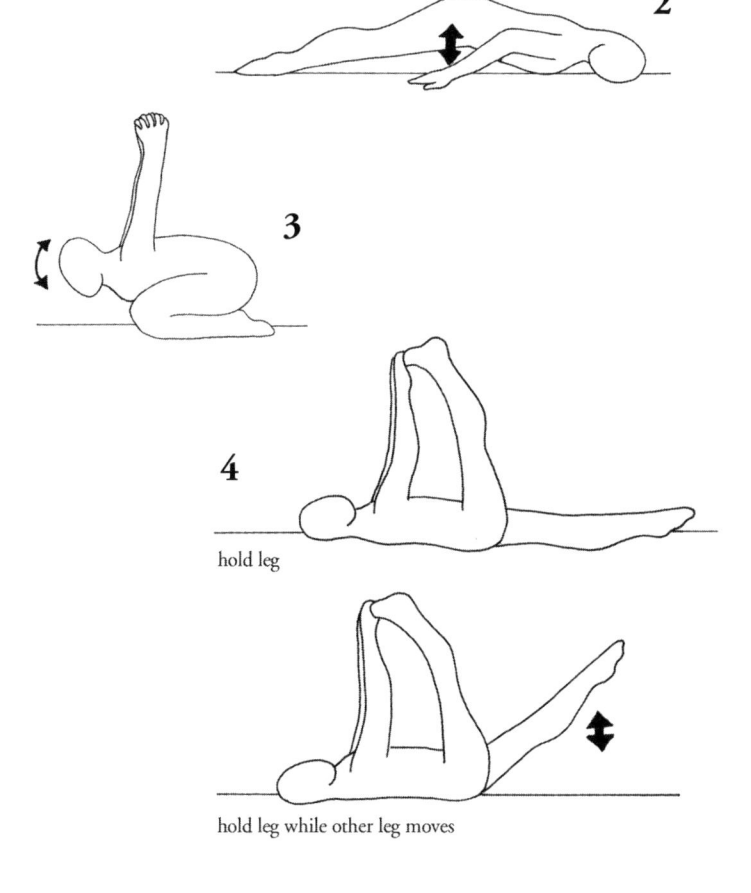

Wake Up the Body to Handle Stress and Strain

October 19, 1988

Simple things to do in bed before you get up for the day.

1. While lying on your back, begin stretching the body in every possible direction. Move up and down, turn left and right, stretch around, and roll back and forth on your back all within a one-foot area. Continue for 1 Minute.

2. Lie on on your belly and jump like a fish. Jump your belly, chest, thighs, and knees; everything jumps. This exercise stimulates the entire body. It is the best exercise. "Your face has to become red." It is good for the circulation, the digestive system, and the colon. 6 Minutes.

3. Come into Baby Pose and lock your hands at the small of your back. Stretch the arms up and begin quickly moving your head up and down, as if vigorously nodding "yes". This is to release anger and tension (like when you become angry and want to hit your head). Do this for 1 Minute and then rotate your head in a circle for 30 Seconds.

4. Lie on your back and raise your left leg up and hold it with both hands. Keep your knees straight. 30 Seconds. Lower your left leg and raise your right leg and hold it with both hands. 30 Seconds. Keep your right leg up holding it with both hands and begin to move the left leg up and down rapidly raising it to a forty-degree angle and lowering it to the floor. 30 Seconds. Change legs, holding the left leg up and moving the right leg. 30 Seconds. Change legs again, holding the right leg up and moving the left leg. 30 Seconds. Move immediately into the next exercise.

5. Remain on your back and bend your knees, and begin rapidly kicking your buttocks alternately with your heels. "Hit hard!" 1 Minute.

6. Come into Cobra Pose, open your eyes wide, stick your tongue out and begin a powerful Lion Breath through your mouth. 1 1/2 Minutes.

If a person in the morning does not move his body in such a way that the capacity of his body, developed during his sleeping hours, is not activated to take the stress and strain of the day then we are getting right straight into a problem for the whole day. We will feel we are awake, that we are perfect, that we can deal with it, bah, bah, bah, but it doesn't work out that way.

Yogi Bhajan

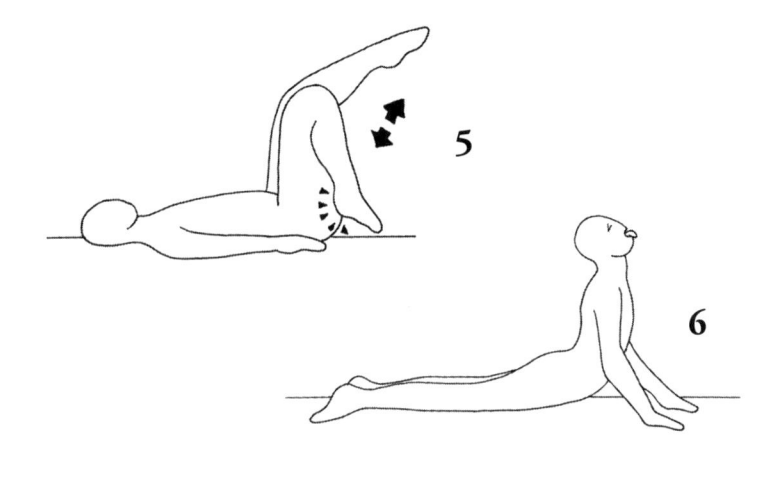

hold leg

hold leg while other leg moves

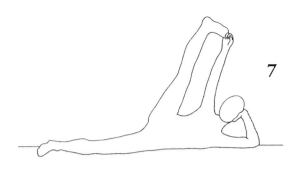

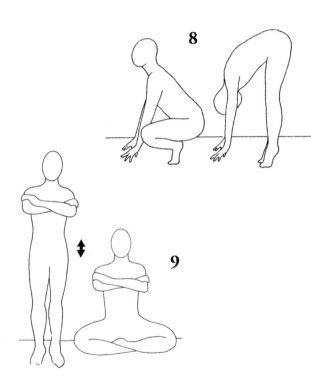

7. Lie on your left side and bring your right leg up straight and hold it with your right hand. 1 Minute. Change sides and hold the left leg up for 30 Seconds.

8. Come into Frog Pose and do 52 frogs. (One count = 1-2 seconds.)

9. Stand up, lock your arms over your chest, holding opposite elbows. Begin moving quickly from the standing position to sitting down on your buttocks and back to standing position, keeping your arms locked. "Get up by your own force." 21 Times. (approximately 3 1/2 minutes) "This stimulates your own magnetic field...no other exercise is equal to it."

10. Lie down in Corpse Pose and deeply relax and sleep to meditative music for 16 Minutes. Then wake up by rolling your hands and feet a few times.

11. Repeat exercise #1 , lying on your back and stretching and moving in all possible directions for 1 Minute. "This time do (it) rhythmically." (Meditative music continues to play.)

12. Repeat exercise #2, lie on your belly and jump like a fish for 1 Minute. (Meditative music continues to play.)

13. Sit up in Easy Pose like a yogi and sing "Dhan Dhan Ram Das Gur" (see page 49). 6 1/2 minutes. Sangeet Kaur's version was played in class. Then deeply inhale and exhale, inhale and exhale, inhale and hold 20 Seconds. Exhale. Inhale and hold 20 seconds. Exhale. Inhale and hold 20 seconds. Exhale and relax the breath.

For Unknown Cause of Sickness

November 7, 1984

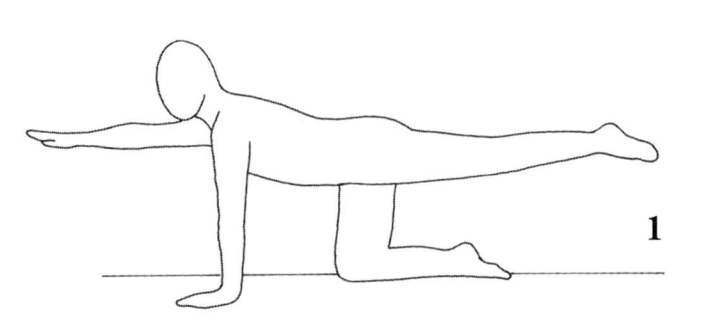

1

1. Be on your hands and knees in Cow Pose and raise the left leg up and raise the right arm up straight in front. "Balance yourself." This posture will balance the body and strengthen the apanic energy. 3 Minutes. Change sides: raise the opposite arm and leg. "Body shakes. It is the navel point adjusting itself." 2 1/2 Minutes. Relax.

2. Stand on your knees and put your arms up straight over your head. Bend backward from the navel and move your arms and neck in a circle; your upper shoulders will move but your knees will not move. This is called "Sobagni Kriya", the kriya of virtue. "Move your upper shoulders, they are very important." 2 Minutes.

3. Sit down and stretch your legs out straight. Grab the soles of your feet and bring your chin between your legs. Hold 2 1/2 Minutes. (At this point Yogi Bhajan began to play the gong.) Remain in the position and concentrate at your third eye for 2 1/2 Minutes more.

4. Lie on your back and, starting from your feet, move your attention up your body, deeply relaxing every part while you project your energy out of your third eye. 6 minutes. (Yogi Bhajan continued to play the gong during this meditative relaxation.)

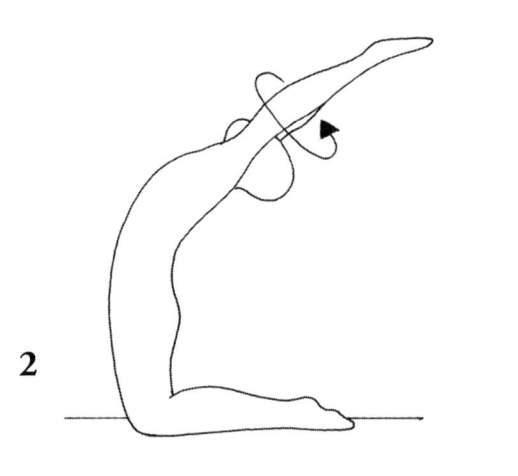

2

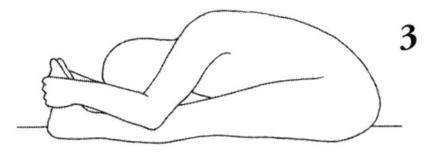

3

Whenever the apaana is not working, even if praana is perfect, you do not act right. Doesn't matter how intelligent you are. Locks in the praanic energy are very, very valid, but locks in the apaanic energy are very subtle... If you cannot balance your body (in exercise #1) it means that your apaanic shakti, the eliminating power which takes away what you don't need, is not in balance. It is weaker.

Yogi Bhajan

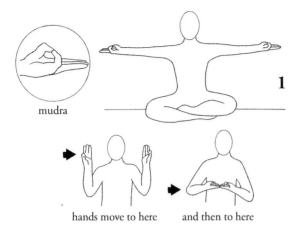

mudra

hands move to here   and then to here

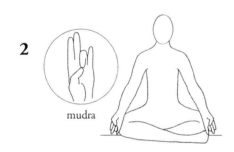

mudra

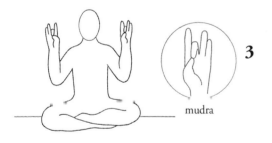

mudra

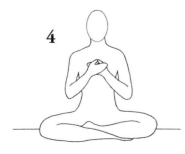

Balancing the Pineal, Pituitary and Hypothalamus

March 13, 1985

"These three mantras and these three kriyas are for the trinity of your soul. It will give you the balance of the hypothalamus, pituitary, and pineal."

1. Sit in Easy Pose with your spine straight. Stretch your arms out straight to the sides parallel to the ground, palms up. Touch the Mercury (pinkie) finger to the thumb, keeping the other fingers straight. Chant the Guru Gaitri Mantra: Gobinde, Mukande, Udaare, Apaare, Hariang, Kariang, Nirnaame, Akaame. (One repetition of the mantra = 10 seconds) 6 Minutes.

To finish: inhale hold the breath 5 seconds and exhale. Then bend elbows bringing the mudra up near the level of the ears and hold for 5 Seconds and then bring the mudra to diaphragm level with the extended fingertips touching and hold for 2 Seconds. Inhale and relax. Twist left and right briefly to "let the energy stimulate in body."

2. Sit in Easy Pose with your thumb touching the Sun (ring) finger, mudra resting on your knees. Chant the Mul Mantra: Ek Ong Kaar, Sat Naam, Kartaa Purkh, Nirbhao, Nirvair, Akaal Moort, Ajoonee, Sai Bhang, Gur Prasaad. Jap. Aad Sach, Jugaad Sach, Hebi Sach, Naanak Hosi Bi Sach. 7 1/2 Minutes. (One repetition of the mantra = 25 seconds.) Inhale and hold the breath for 20 Seconds. Relax. Then "give your energy to every organ" by twisting left and right and moving around for about 30 Seconds.

3. Remain in Easy Pose. Touch the Saturn (middle) finger and thumb and bring the mudra up to the level of the ears, elbows bent. Chant the Guru Gaitri Mantra (same as in #1.) 3 1/2 Minutes. Inhale, hold 15-20 seconds, Exhale. Relax. Stretch briefly to loosen your muscles.

4. Still sitting in easy pose, place the hands on the chest at the heart center, right hand over left, thumbs touching. Chant in a monotone:

Har Har Gobinde, Har Har Mukande /repeat this line 3 times. (3 times = 12 seconds)
Har Har Udaare, Har Har Apaare /repeat this line 3 times.
Har Har Hariang, Har Har Kariang /repeat this line 3 times.
Har Har Nirnaame, Har Har Akaame /repeat this line 3 times.

2 1/2 Minutes.

Our system has what is called a 'reserve force.' It is a meditating power that is the cooperation among the hypothalamus, pituitary, and pineal. Medical science has not totally understood it, neither has it reached it. The body mechanism is under the control of this trinity: pineal is called the father, pituitary is called the son, and hypothalamus is called the holy ghost. It is called the trinity of the life psyche. Kundalini Yoga is a simple methodical system to reach that reserve of the psyche through which we can live and develop forever.

Yogi Bhajan

19
Owner's Manual

Optimum Health

October 5, 1988

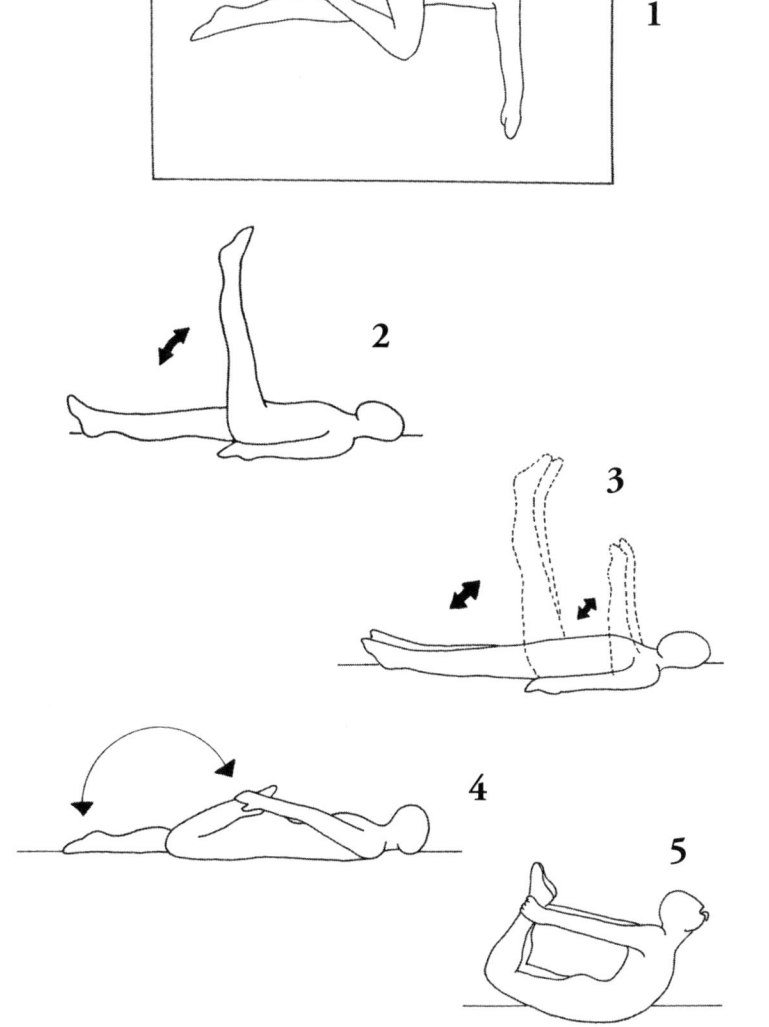

1. Lying on your back, bend your right knee and bring it across your body to the left side in a cat stretch. Your shoulders remain on the floor. Cat stretch to the left side and then to the right side 21 times on each side.

2. Still lying on your back, begin alternate leg lifts. Lift your left leg to 90 degrees and lower it. Then raise your right leg to 90 degrees and lower it. Let the legs "hammer" the ground. Continue rapid alternate leg lifts for 1 1/2 Minutes.

3. Still lying on your back simultaneously raise both arms and legs up to 90 degrees and then lower them and raise them again. Move quickly. 2 Minutes.

4. Lying on your stomach reach back and grab your left ankle and pull the left leg down towards the left buttock. Then release the left ankle and grab the right ankle and stretch it down towards the right buttock. Continue alternating the stretch for 1 Minute.

5. Continue lying on your stomach, grab both ankles and come up into Bow Pose. Roll on your stomach back and forth like a hobby horse, extend your tongue out of your mouth and do Breath of Fire through your mouth.
1 1/2 Minutes. Let the body open up.

6. Roll quickly onto your back and begin jumping your whole body up and down. 2 Minutes.

7. Come into Cobra Pose and begin moving up and down from Cobra Pose; alternate between lying on your stomach on the floor and being up in Cobra Pose. Stick your tongue all the way out and breathe through your mouth. Do 52 Cobra lifts. (1 Cobra lift = 2 seconds)

When you say nothing, do nothing, be nothing, then you are a lighthouse. Nobody can wreck near you. This is the one thing in life you have to do. Spread the light. Be the lighthouse.

Yogi Bhajan

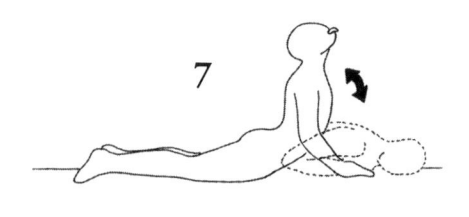

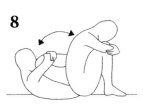

8

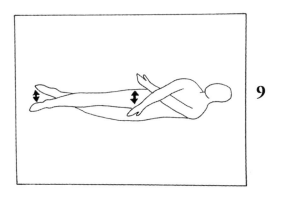

9

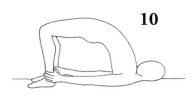

10

8. Lie on your back, bend your knees and hug them to your chest with your arms. Put your nose between your knees and rock forward and back on your spine. "Roll up and down, just like a roller coaster, all the way." 2 Minutes.
(1 spinal roll = 4 seconds)

9. Lie flat on your back and begin criss-crossing your arms and legs rapidly back and forth. 2 Minutes.

10. Still lying on your back, come into a variation of Half Wheel Pose by grabbing your ankles and arching your spine, while still resting your shoulders and head on the floor. Go to sleep in this posture while listening to relaxing meditative music. 7 Minutes.

11. Turn onto your belly and sleep for another 8 minutes. Meditative music continues.

12. Jump from your stomach onto your back in one quick move and take a nap. 11 Minutes. "Guru Ram Das Lullaby" was played in class.

13. Roll your hands and feet (30 seconds) and do cat stretches (30 seconds). Wake yourself up. Then rise up slowly and sit like a yogi.

14. The following meditation was done to the version of "Wahe Guru, Wahe Guru, Wahe Guru, Wahe Jio" by Bhai Avtar Singh and Bhai Gurucharn Singh: Sit in Easy Pose, with your eyes closed, looking at the tip of your nose from the inside, through your closed eyes. 3 1/2 Minutes. Still in Easy Pose with your eyes closed, change your focus to the top of your head. 4 Minutes. (Yogi Bhajan played the gong for this part.)

To finish: inhale and exhale quickly two times, then stretch, wake up, and relax.

21

Yoga for Circulation and Energy

September 28, 1988

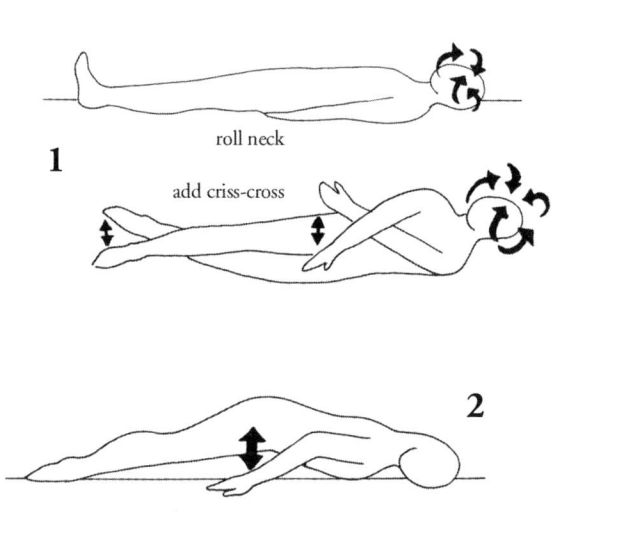

roll neck

add criss-cross

The navel point is the source of the purity, the energy, the divinity.

Yogi Bhajan

1. Lie down on your back with your legs out straight and your hands under your buttocks. Begin to roll your neck in all directions while you relax your body. Roll it any way you can, but keep the rest of the body relaxed. After 2 1/2 Minutes, begin to criss-cross your arms and your legs while continuing to roll your neck in all directions. Make your movements heavy and fast. Coordinate the rhythm of the neck, arm, and leg movements, so that the breath automatically becomes Breath of Fire. 4 Minutes. This exercise strengthens the immune system.

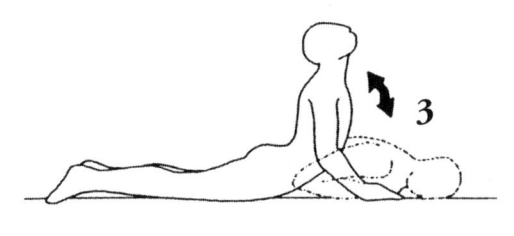

2. Lie on your stomach with your arms at your sides and your hands on the ground. Beat your belly on the ground, jumping all the way up to your shoulders. "Lift and hit...quick, fast, heavy...Get rid of all the anxiety." 2 1/2 Minutes.

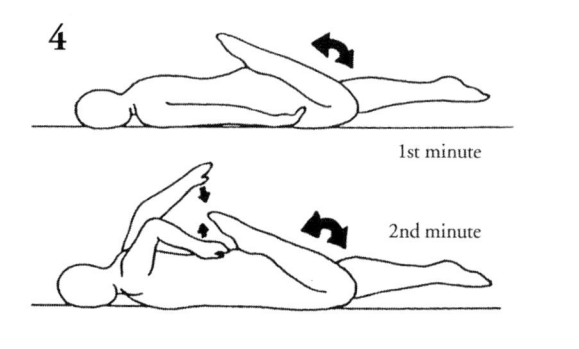

3. Come into Cobra Pose and then touch your forehead to the ground and rise back up into Cobra Pose again. Move quickly. 1 Minute.

4. Lie flat on your belly and begin to kick your buttocks with alternate heels and also to kick the ground as you bring your feet down, so that there is impact at both ends of the action. 1 Minute. Then begin using your palms to softly hit the kidney points in the small of the back as you continue your rhythmic kicking motion. This will stimulate both the digestive system and the kidneys. 1 Minute.

1st minute

2nd minute

5. Lie on your back and jump your body vigorously like a jumping fish. 2 Minutes. This will adjust the electromagnetic field of the nervous system.

6. Wrap your arms around your knees and press them hard against your chest, while lying on your back. Make your body more and more tense until it is as hard as a stone. 1 Minute. In the same posture raise your nose to your knees and loudly sing along with Livtar Singh's version of "I am Thine". 2 Minutes. The words of this mantra are for your radiant body: Hummee Humm, Toomee Toom, Wahe Guroo, I am Thine, in mine, myself, Wahe Guroo.

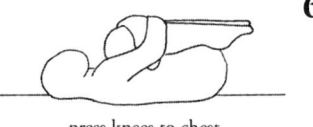

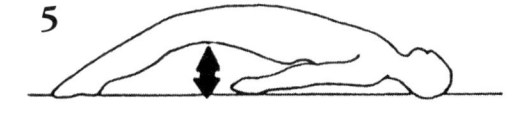

press knees to chest

nose to knees & sing

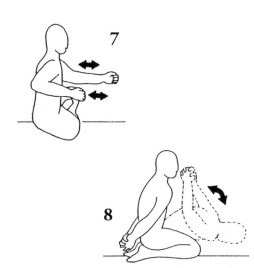

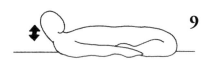

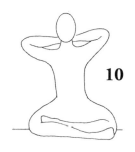

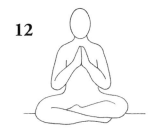

Inhale deeply and rise up.

7. In Easy Pose, makes fists and begin punching powerfully with Breath of Fire. Hard and fast. 1 1/2 Minutes.

8. Sit on your heels. Join your hands together behind your back, fingers interlocked and arms straight and stretched. As you listen to Ragi Sat Nam Singh's version of "Jaap Sahib" bow forward to bring your forehead to the floor and raise your arms straight up behind you each time he sings "Namo" or "Namastang" and then return to your upright position. 4 1/2 Minutes. Only move on "namo" or "namastang," the rest of the time you do not move.

9. Sit on your heels, then spread your heels apart so that you are sitting between them (Celibate Pose). Hold the position for 30 seconds then lie back so that your upper torso is on the floor. Start once again at the beginning of Ragi Sat Nam Singh's "Jaap Sahib" and raise your head up off the floor and lie back down each time he chants "Namo" or "Namastang." 3 1/2 Minutes. Yogis say that a person should be in a position to comfortably sit in this posture unless there is some difficulty with the sex glands or immune system.

10. Sit in Easy Pose for 30 seconds then lock your hands behind your head for another 30 seconds. Maintain the posture as you listen to Bhai Avtar Singh's "Jai Te Gung," pulling and releasing the root lock each time you hear the word "Jai." Meditate on the energy from your navel to the top of your head. 5 1/2 Minutes.

11. Lie on your back and go quickly into a deep nap. Relax your body and relax your mind. Relate to your soul. (Yogi Bhajan played "Guru Ram Das Lullaby" during this relaxation.) After 7 Minutes, take some time to gracefully wake up your body: stretch, do cat stretch, and roll your feet and hands.

12. Slowly rise up into Easy Pose while singing along with Sangeet Kaur's "Dhan Dhan Ram Das Gur" with your hands in prayer pose at your heart center. Press your hands strongly against each other to balance the energy and sing loudly. 10 1/2 Minutes.

To finish: Inhale long and deeply (approximately 10 second inhale) and exhale completely. Do this breath three times.

23

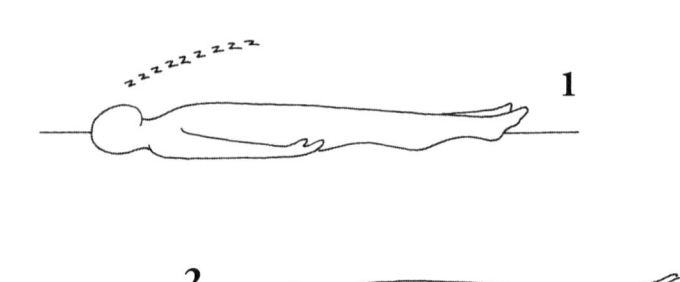

To Relieve Inner Anger

September 21, 1988

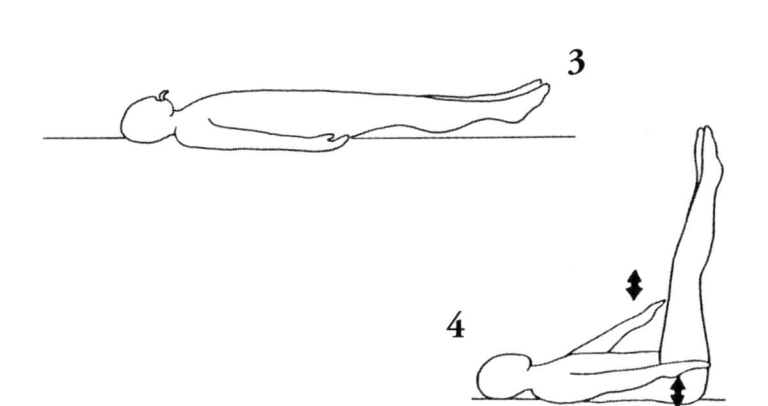

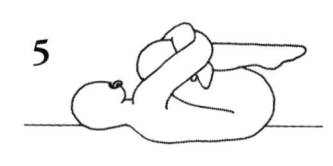

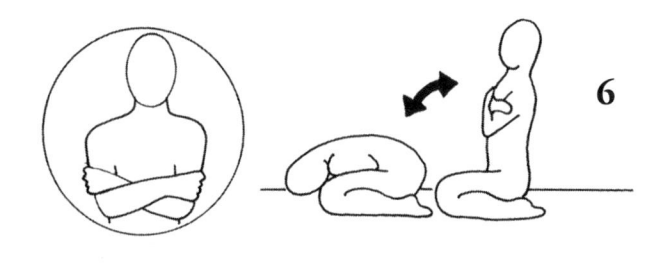

1. Lie down flat on your back in a relaxed posture with your arms at your sides, palms up and your legs slightly apart. Pretend to snore. "You think snoring is a nasty thing. It is not. It will relax you right there." 1 Minute.

2. Still lying on your back, keeping your legs out straight, raise both legs up to 6 inches and hold. 2 Minutes. This exercise balances anger. It pressurizes the navel to balance the entire system. In this posture you will become angry within about forty-five seconds.

3. Remaining in the posture with your legs up at 6 inches, stick your big lion tongue out and do Breath of Fire through your mouth. 1 1/2 Minutes.

4. Still lying on your back, lift your legs up to 90 degrees with your arms on the ground by your sides. Begin to beat the ground with your hands using all the anger you can achieve. Beat hard and fast. Get the anger out! 2 Minutes.

5. Still on your back, use your arms to press your knees tightly against your chest, and stick your tongue out. Inhale through your open mouth and exhale through your nose. 2 minutes. This is Bhajar (stone) Praanayam. It can make even a stone-head think right.

6. Sit in Celibate Pose, buttocks on the floor between the heels. Cross your arms over your chest and press them hard against your rib cage, making your rib cage like stone. (This is Bhajar Bhand, the stone lock.) Bend forward and touch your forehead to the floor as if you are bowing. For 2 Minutes move at a pace of approximately 30 bows per minute, then for another 30 Seconds speed up and move as fast as you can. (2 1/2 Minutes total time)

7. Sitting with your legs straight out in front of you, begin to beat every part of your body with your open palms. "Hit hard." Leave no spot untouched. It's a free massage. Move fast. 2 Minutes.

When the inverted anger becomes part of the body, the simple effect is that you have absolutely no relationship with your Self... Inferiority complex or superiority complex are a cover-up of inner anger. Manipulation and lying is part of inner anger. Not being self-sustaining or having a foundation to work it out is an inner anger. All skin diseases are inner anger. Misbehavior, wrong calculation, self-destruction, destroying the business, destroying the relationship are all inner anger...On the other hand, anger comes from the place of the Agaan Granthi. It is the area of the heart, it is the blood, it is the circulation, it is the diaphragm,

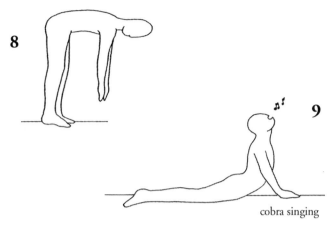

8

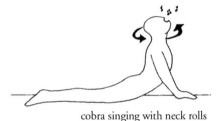

cobra singing

9

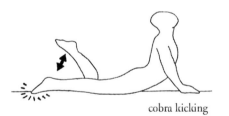

cobra singing with neck rolls

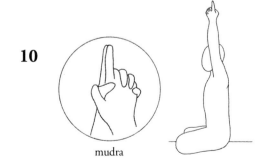

cobra kicking

10

mudra

8. Stand up. Bend forward, keeping your back parallel to the ground, and let your arms and hands hang loose. Remain in this posture and sing a mantra for 3 Minutes. This is called "forced circulation." If you get dizzy in this posture, sit down immediately. (In class, Yogi Bhajan played a tape of "Guru, Guru, Wahe Guru, Guru Ram Das Guru.")

9. Continue singing as you come into Cobra Pose, keeping the elbows straight and stretching the spine. Sing from the navel. 1 Minute. Then begin circling your neck, continue to sing. 30 Seconds. Stay in Cobra Pose and begin kicking the ground with alternate feet. 30 Seconds.

10. Sit in Easy Pose and close your eyes. Stretch your arms over your head, keeping the elbows straight, and interlock your fingers, with the index fingers pointing straight up. Begin Sat Kriya for 1 1/2 Minutes.

11. Lie down on your back and nap for 11 Minutes. Quickly get deeply into your relaxation. Yogi Bhajan played the gong.

To come back from the layout, rotate your hands and feet. Cat stretch left and right. Tense up your body briefly and then shake every part of your body.

(Note: In class there was an interlude between exercise #10 and the layout when Yogi Bhajan had two students lead the class in Celestial Communication for six minutes and then the class took the five minute nap.)

it is the heart pumping. Blah, blah. The whole life depends on it. So it is the center of the heart, it is the furnace. Either it can cook for you or it can burn down your house and there is nothing in between. That is the tragedy of it.

Yogi Bhajan

Give Power To The Brain

May 29, 1985

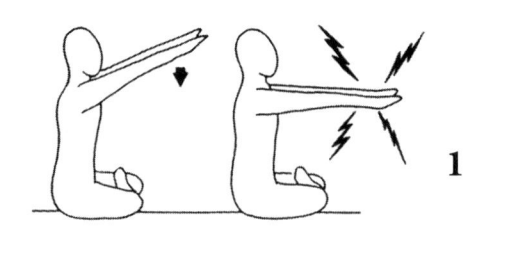

"Today every exercise we are going to do is with the elbows and with the hands. We are not going to touch anything else."

1. Sit in Easy Pose with arms together in front of the body up at about a 45 degree angle with the palms facing down. Rapidly push the arms down from this position with full force until they are a little below parallel with the ground and then return them up to about 45 degrees. The arms are stiff and straight and the movement is very quick, "with the force of lightning." The eyes are focused straight ahead and, if you do it right, the breath will be automatically regulated after four or five movements. Continue 4 1/2 Minutes then inhale and hold the breath briefly and then relax.

The stiffness of the hands and the power of the hands is to create a special breath called Shakti Shallee Praanayam, lightning breath. It's a very sacred way of recharging your entire inner being.

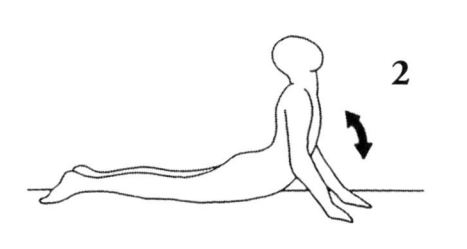

2. Rise up into Cobra Pose and then rapidly lower your torso back down touching the tip of your nose to the floor and then return to Cobra Pose. Just *touch* your nose, don't hit it on the floor. Although this is a quick movement, come up into a full Cobra Pose with the elbows straight.
3 1/2 Minutes.

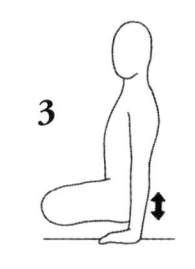

3. Sit in Lotus Pose or Easy Pose. Place your hands on the floor on either side of the hips. Lift the body up off the ground and let it drop. Continue 2 1/2 Minutes. "Musical butts, they call it."

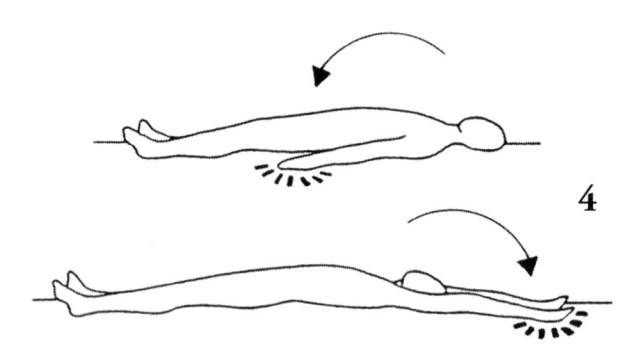

4. Lie on your back with your arms straight out on the floor overhead. With the arms stiff and straight, bring them forward and hit the floor on either side of the hips with the palms of the hands. Then bring the arms back over the head hitting the floor with the back of the hands. Hit the ground with equal force each time. Move very fast. 1 1/2 Minutes.

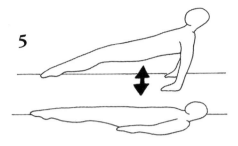

5

5. Rise up into Back Platform Pose, then lower the body back down to the floor and then return to Back Platform Pose. Continue for 4 Minutes. "It is just like a wave of the body." Correctly doing this movement can bring relaxation to the ovaries.

6. Rise up into Front Platform Pose and lower the body flat to the floor and then return to Front Platform Pose. 1 1/2 Minutes.

7. Relax the posture and lie on your stomach for 13 minutes. Relax and listen to meditative music. Keep your arms along the sides of your body. (Yogi Bhajan played the gong while the meditative music was also playing.)

8. Slowly rise up to sitting and move the body slowly and sinuously, loosening up every muscle, while listening to meditative music. It is a free-flowing movement. "The body needs this healing energy at this time." 7 1/2 Minutes. (Yogi Bhajan played the gong.)

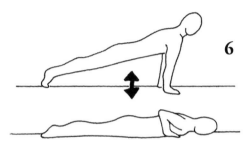

6

27

For the Left and Right Hemispheres of the Brain

May 7, 1986

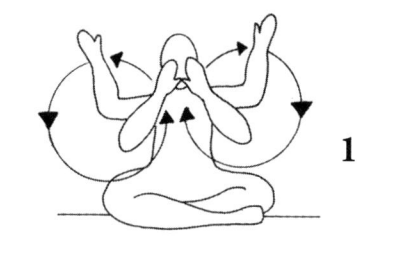

1

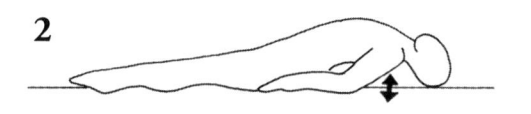

2

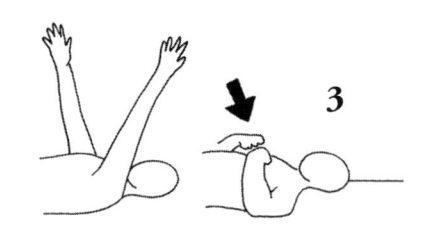

3

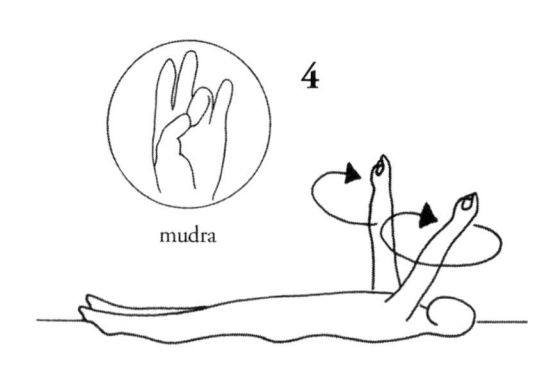

mudra

4

This set works on the shoulders. "These are very high class mudras...exercises as old as the Aryans. This was their morning wake-up."

1. Sit in Easy Pose, elbows bent, with the upper arms parallel to the ground, the lower arms angled slightly forward with the palms facing forward. Moving just from the shoulders, circle your arms in outward circles, moving down with the speed and force of a "thundering bird (120 mph)." As the hands come in and up and pass the level of the chin/nose, the thumbs lightly touch. "The downward speed is so heavy that you must automatically go upward. If you use any strength going upward, it means that your downward speed is not correct." Use both arms with equal force. Rotate your shoulder muscles. Your breath will change and it will open up your lungs. 6 1/2 Minutes. "Just see if your brain is connected to your lymph glands or not."

2. Lie down flat on your back and "jump" your shoulders. Jumping means to quickly move the entire area from the lower spine to the upper shoulders up and down. 3 1/2 Minutes. Allow the movement to massage your ribcage, relax and give relief to your heart muscles, and relieve tension in the neck, lower back, and arms.

3. Still lying on your back, lift your arms straight up, and then angle them out to the sides at about a 45 degree angle to the body. Your fingers are open wide when the arms are out. Close your hands tightly into fists and forcefully bring the hands toward the chest stopping just about an inch before the fists touch the chest. "Hit hard, touch it not." Then let the momentum of the movement automatically bounce the hands back to the starting position with the palms open and the fingers spread wide. Pull your arms in powerfully, but don't touch your chest. Move with the speed of the first exercise. Continue 2 Minutes.

4. Still on your back, raise your arms straight up perpendicular to the floor. Put your hands in "Surya Mudra" with the thumbs and Sun (ring) fingers touching. Keep the arms straight and rapidly circle them in large circles moving from the shoulders. 1 1/2 Minutes.

We all have problems here and there. And every problem in our life has a solution. When we consider that our problems have no solutions, then we start going to the psychics and astrologers and all that. And I have seen that fun part. But if you really want to know, the psyche of life is nothing but a simple challenge. We can create the balance in our own psyche whenever we feel like.

Yogi Bhajan

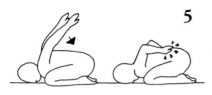

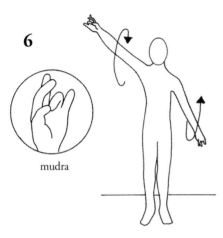

mudra

5. Come into Baby Pose and raise your arms up as high as possible behind your back. The top shoulder muscle must move, don't just move from the elbows. With the palms open, hit the lower back simultaneously with both hands, using the whole arm. Raise the arms again and repeat. Hit hard, creating a sound. 4 1/2 Minutes. "Give yourself a heavy massage."

6. Stand up. Make a mudra with the thumbs and Sun (ring) fingers touching and with the first two fingers crossed. Start with one arm up and one arm down and circle the arms backward, maintaining the relationship between the arms. No bend in the elbows. Move fast, like an airplane propeller. 3 1/2 Minutes. (This exercise was done to Singh Kaur's "Har Har Gobinday." Three revolutions of the arms = 6 seconds.)

7. Lie down, relax, and go to sleep. Yogi Bhajan played the gong and various meditative songs. At 9 1/2 Minutes, he instructed the class to sing along with Guru Dass Singh's recording of "Flowers in the Rain" for the last 1 1/2 Minutes of the relaxation, then had them roll their hands and feet and come sitting up as they continued to sing for another 2 1/2 Minutes.

For Mental Balance

October 16, 1985

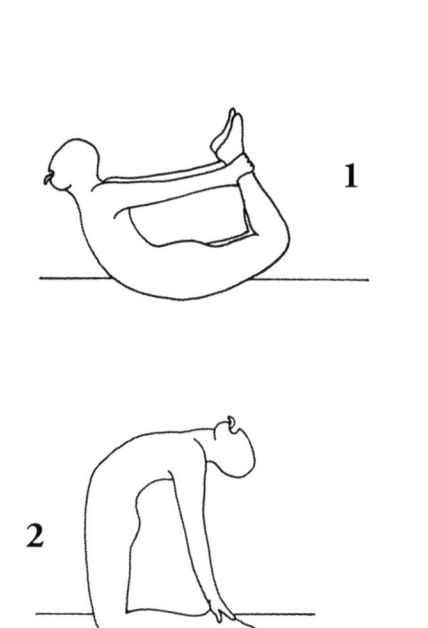

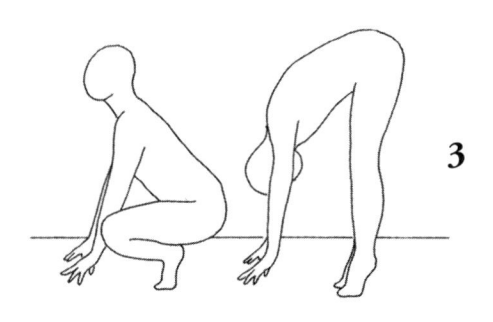

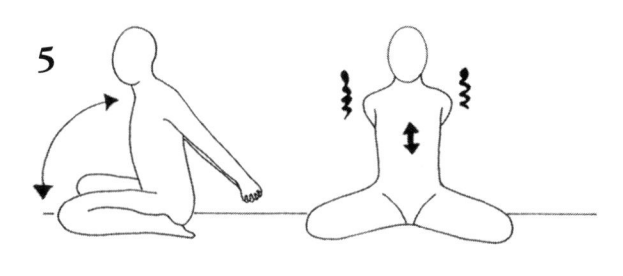

1. Bow Pose: lying on your stomach, reach back grabbing your ankles and arch your body up like a bow. "Pull the muscles of the thigh to a corrective point that they can react with the body." After 2 Minutes stick out your tongue as far as possible and breathe heavily through your mouth. (This is Singha Praanayam, the "breath of the lion." The taste of the tongue will change after a few seconds.) Continue for 1 1/2 Minutes more. Yogis believe that pain in the thigh muscles during these exercises indicates that the levels of potassium and magnesium are off and that the mental health is not in good shape.

2. Camel Pose: from a sitting position on your heels, rise up onto your knees. Tuck your tailbone under to keep your pelvic bone stable and aligned over your knees. Lift your heart up and lengthen your spine. Reach back to grab your ankles or your heels. Allow your head to drop backwards. Stick out your tongue as far as possible and begin the "Breath of the Lion." 1 1/2 Minutes.

3. Frog Pose: squat down, balancing on the balls of your feet, your heels are off the ground but touching each other. Place your fingertips on the ground between the feet. Your head faces forward. Inhale and straighten your legs, raising the buttocks high while keeping your heels off the ground. (The head moves toward knees while the fingertips stay on the ground.) On the exhale return to the squatting position. Continue for a total of 108 Frogs. In class, the students counted aloud from 1 to 108. (Approximately 2 minutes) "This exercise straightens out the mind in a couple of minutes."

4. Relax in Easy Pose for 11 Minutes.

5. Celibate Pose Variation: from a sitting position on your heels move your heels out to the sides so that your buttocks are resting on the floor. Spread your knees as far apart as possible. Clasp your hands behind your back. From this position lower your torso forward to the floor and rise back up, moving your shoulders from side to side weaving "like a snake." Continue this up-and-down-torso and side-to-side-shoulder movements for 3 Minutes. Dance your spine.

Faith is your essence. Deal with your faith faithfully. Otherwise you will end up with filth.

Yogi Bhajan

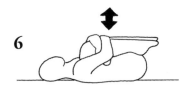

6

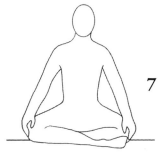

7

6. Lie on your back, bring your knees to your chest and lock your arms around your knees. While holding yourself in this position, bounce your body up and down on the floor. 7 Minutes. Keep the arms locked tight. "Keep the hand lock perfect...and try to free yourself." (When you have a sexual imbalance, your mood is always off and you act crazy or depressed, yogis advise that three minutes of this exercise can bring you back to normal.)

7. "Nar Narayan Kriya." Sit up like a yogi in Easy Pose with your spine straight and your hands resting on your knees. Inhale and powerfully exhale the breath in one stroke so that the sound of the breath leaving the nostrils sounds like "Har." (Exhale one "Har" per second.) Pump the navel so that the exhalation goes from the navel to the nostrils. Create the sound "Har" with the tip of the nostrils. The rib cage will lift with the power of the breath. 3 to 5 Minutes.

"Stimulate the Ida and Pingala at the tip of the nose. Build the divine breath, the praanic breath, the basic breath."

8. Relax on your back and nap. 8 Minutes. (Yogi Bhajan played the gong.)

To finish: move around, still on your back, wiggling like a fish. Move all of your muscles Dance while lying down. 4 Minutes. (In class Yogi Bhajan played Sangeet Kaur's recording of "Naad, the Blessing".)

NOTE: Yogi Bhajan said that by regularly practicing exercises 1 and 2 for 3 minutes each and then doing 108 Frog Poses you can achieve physical and mental health. (For this purpose, all three exercises are to be done with the tongue extended and "the breath of the lion." He noted that he did not teach exercise #3 with Breath of the Lion in class because the class was not yet ready for it.)

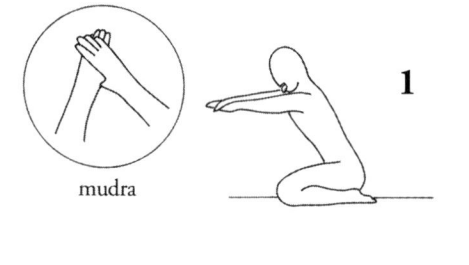

mudra

1

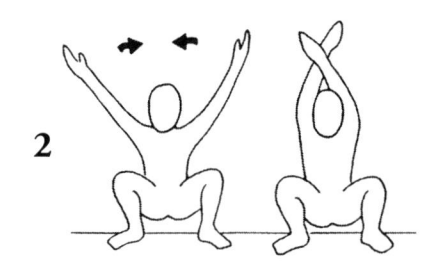

2

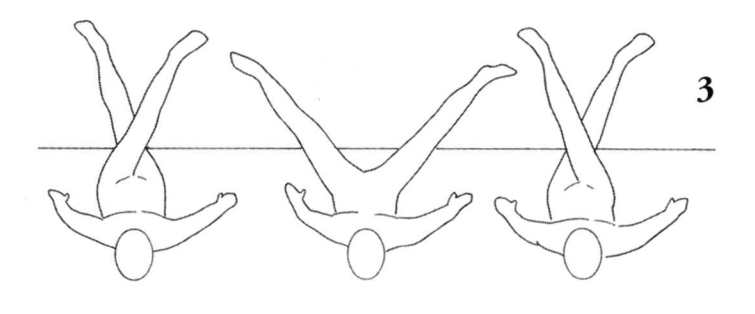

3

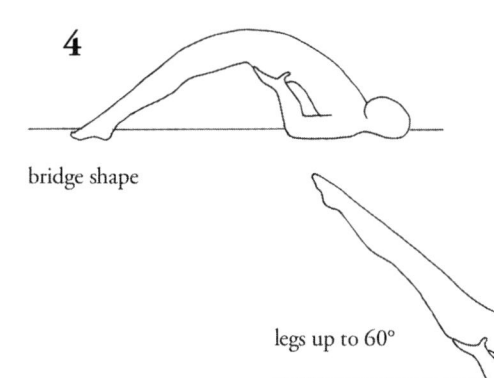

4

bridge shape

legs up to 60°

To Take Away Stress

March 28, 1987

This set is designed to take away stress so we can totally enjoy what we are living for.

1. Sit on your heels, arms stretched out in front, right hand over left, with the thumbs locked. (When Yogi Bhajan demonstrated this mudra, the right hand was over the left, palms down, and the left thumb locked the right thumb against the left palm.) Lean the torso forward 60 degrees. This angle is very important. "It's an angle which will keep such a balance that your body will become hard like steel...You will totally vitalize the entire body and the energy to one-ness." Keep your arms straight and parallel to the floor, stretching forward as far as you can. 2 Minutes. Maintain the stretch, put out your tongue, and do Breath of Fire through the open mouth. This breath adds extra strength to your nervous system. 1 1/2 Minutes.

2. Sit in Crow Pose and stretch your arms up and out in a "V". Begin clapping your hands over your head as fast as you can, moving the entire arm from the shoulder. 30 Seconds. Then continue the motion, but instead of clapping, criss-cross the arms over your head. The palms face each other as if they were clapping but they do not touch. This gives the mind basic strength and balances the nervous system. (Try to feel negative or depressed in this posture, you won't be able to do it.) 3 Minutes.

3. Lie flat on your back, raise legs up to 90 degrees and begin criss-crossing the legs as fast as possible. If you do it slowly, it won't work. Keep your legs straight. "It's going to go right into your guts." This exercise adjusts the sexual area. 3 Minutes.

4. Lie on your back and bring your heels together. Place your hands under your buttocks and arch your hips to create a bridge shape without bending your knees. Keep your shoulders, head, and toes on the ground. Hold for 1 Minute. Using this posture as a base, raise your heels about 3 feet off the ground (to approximately 60 degrees) and hold the position. Your weight will rest on your elbows. 3 Minutes. This exercise brings sexual balance. It can change the grey matter of the brain.

What we know about yoga is very simple: a definite, defined individual, called a human being, can use his mental, spiritual, and physical being to tap into the Infinity of God, or Infinity itself. I do not know whether you believe in God or not. It's a matter of chance... When you believe in God, you believe in Infinity. You believe you can see all goodness in all. And you can see weaknesses in all and you do practice your tolerance and your capacity for tolerance, compassion, and kindness. That's what they are meant for.

Yogi Bhajan

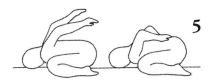

5

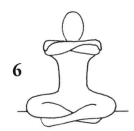

6

5. Sit in Baby Pose and with your hands pat your lower back rhythmically (the area of the 3rd, 4th and 5th vertebrae and the kidney area.) Pat with a slow, relaxing, musical rhythm. 2 1/2 Minutes. Listen to the sound inside you as you pat your back. If done right, this will relax you.

6. Sit in Easy Pose with arms held at chin level in front of the body, right arm on top of left. Lock the hands above opposite elbows, with the fingers on top and the thumbs underneath. The hands have to be tight and the arms have to stay firmly in place. Be as still as a statue. Make absolutely no movement. Straighten your spine, pull in the chin, close your eyes and chant the shabad "Rakhe Rakhan Har" (see page 50). Singh Kaur's version was played in class. 13 Minutes. Consciously use the tip of your tongue on the upper palate when chanting to stimulate the hypothalamus. The words of this shabad are "the best typical electronic signal your hypothalamus can send to the Cosmic Self of the total nebula, Universal Energy."
Inhale, hold briefly, and relax.

7. Lie down in Corpse Pose and relax. Close your eyes and breathe absolutely long and deep. "Tell your ears to hear and yourself to meditate." (Yogi Bhajan played to gong in the rhythm of the three: "the Earth, the space, and the Beyond.")
5 1/2 Minutes.

Wake up sequence. Move briefly through the following actions. Take a deep Cat Stretch left and right as strongly as you can.(30 seconds) Rise up to sitting. Each of the following movements takes 5-10 seconds. Raise and lower your shoulders. Dance them really well. Roll your neck loosely, then open your fingers and stretch your hands like you are grabbing something. Then quickly blink your eyes and move your lips. Roll your tongue around the front of your teeth. Stretch your rib cage from the insides, roll your digestive area, and end by wiggling your toes.

Colon Cleanser

June 3, 1986

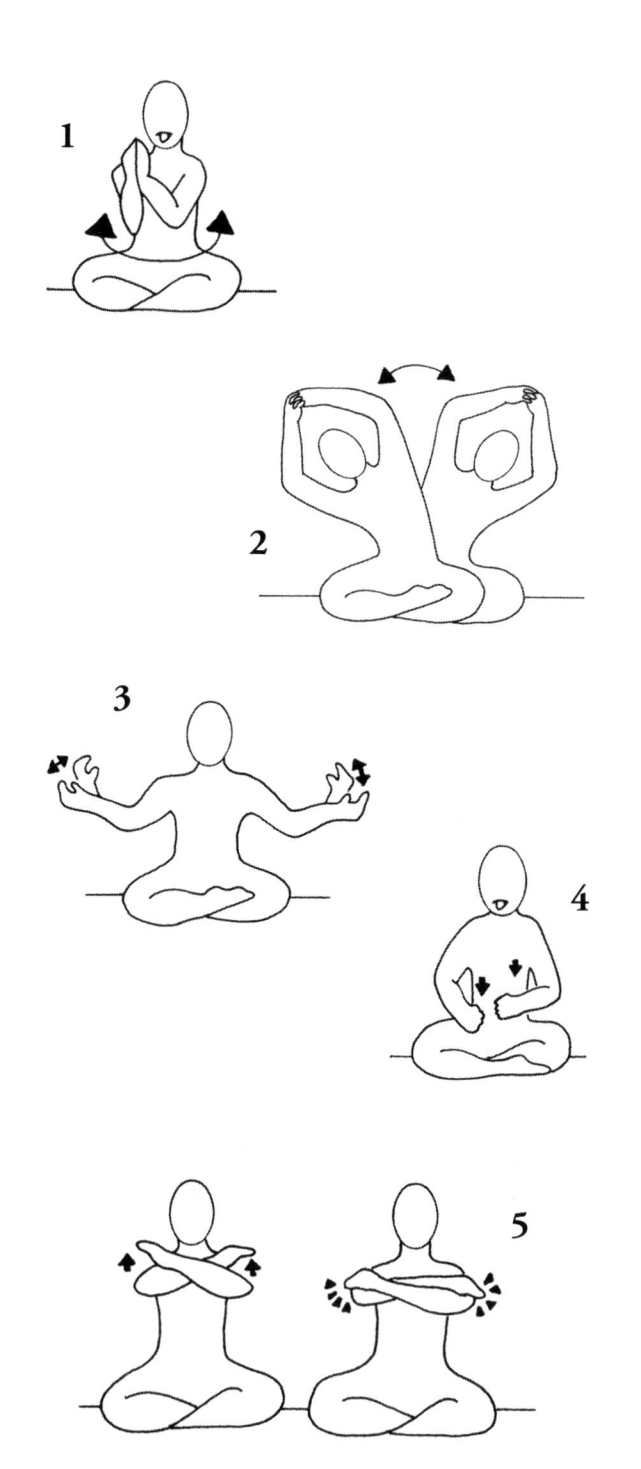

Please have 12 oz. of prune juice with you when you begin the set.

1. Sitting in Easy Pose, bring your hands into Prayer Pose with the thumbs locked over each other on the right side of your body, with the mudra held in front on your right shoulder. (The mudra is held high: the thumbs are a little above the level of your shoulder.) Keeping the arms locked in the position at the right side, the pressure between the arms creates a fulcrum around which the body moves. Twist your spine left and right moving from the lower abdomen. Do Breath of Fire through your open mouth with the tongue out. 6 1/2 Minutes. Correctly done, this exercise will give you a mild sinking sensation of nausea

2. Still in Easy Pose, bring your arms up into an arc over your head, interlace your fingers to lock your hands together with the palms down and lean left and right as far as possible. "Right on the arc line." 5 minutes.

3. Extend both arms out to the sides at a comfortable angle to the body. The elbows are bent and the hands are palms up. The wrists should be very loose and the hands should be very loose and heavy. You should feel the weight of the hands as if they are separate. Begin moving your arms so that the hands loosely flop up and down. Shake the hands by moving the arms. It will straighten your lower spine. 3 Minutes.

4. Remain in Easy Pose, make fists of your hands, and alternately hit the area where your legs join the hips. There is an indentation where "your fists will fit and, if you press, it hurts." Do a powerful Breath of Fire with your mouth open and tongue extended. Move faster and faster. The taste of the tongue will change if you do it correctly.
3 Minutes.

5. Cross your arms over your chest, with your hands holding onto the opposite arm just above the elbow. Hold the arms up so that the elbows are held at shoulder level. Begin raising the forearms from the elbows so that you can hit your palms against your upper arms. Continually move heavier and faster. "It's a perfect balance, it's a dance." 5 Minutes.

We are moving the colon and whatever those little mucousy things it creates. It creates a kind of cone. Colon has an attitude to form cones and that mucousy stuff stops your ability to absorb nutrients. Yogic science says that your health depends on that little thing in the center of your tummy.

Yogi Bhajan

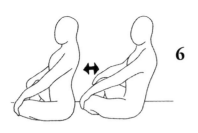

6. Remain in Easy Pose and place your hands on your knees. Begin to flex your spine as fast as you can. Breathe and move powerfully. 1 1/2 Minutes.

7. Open your arms out to the sides so that they are a little higher than parallel to the ground. Rapidly bring them up and cross them in front of your face, keeping the arms completely straight. This criss-cross movement should be very fast. 2 minutes. Inhale and stretch the arms out and exhale. Inhale, hold the breath and pump the navel for 15 seconds. Exhale. Inhale and repeat the navel pump. Relax and drink all of your prune juice.

(In class there was an interlude of about four minutes while the students drank their juice.)

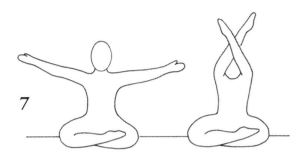

8. To press the prune juice out of your stomach: in Easy Pose, swing your arms up and to the left, twisting the torso to the left as you do so, hold the position for 1 second. Then swing the arms down diagonally to the right, twisting the body to the right side and hold the position for 1 second. (Your torso moves with your arms as they move diagonally up to the left and down to the right.) Continue for 1 Minute.

9. Lock your arms over your chest with your palms holding just above the elbows of the opposite arms. Be calm, quiet, and peaceful. Create a slow rhythmic pumping of the navel to the beat of Livtar Singh Khalsa's recording of "I Am Thine in Mine Myself." Meditate silently pumping the navel for 4 1/2 Minutes and then, continue to pump the navel and sing along for another 3 Minutes.

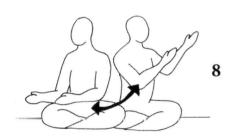

10. Come into Baby Pose. Meditate to Jasbir Kaur's recording of the "Mool Mantra" (Yogi Bhajan played the gong). After 7 1/2 Minutes slowly and gradually rise up. Put your legs out straight in front. Stretch forward to grab your toes 3 times. Then roll your head and neck in a figure eight. 30 Seconds. Come into a steady meditative posture and meditatively relax to soothing spiritual music. 11 Minutes.

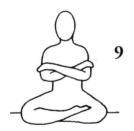

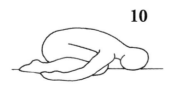

Maintain the Spleen

October 17, 1984

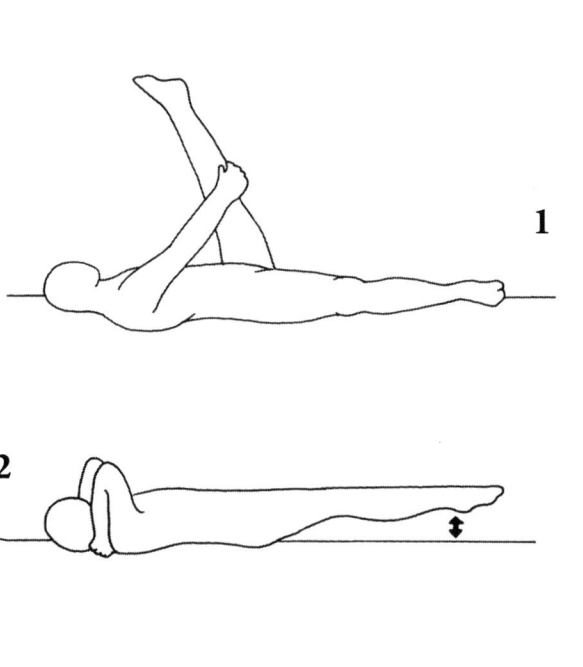

1

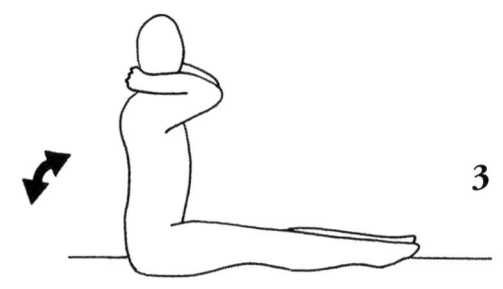

2

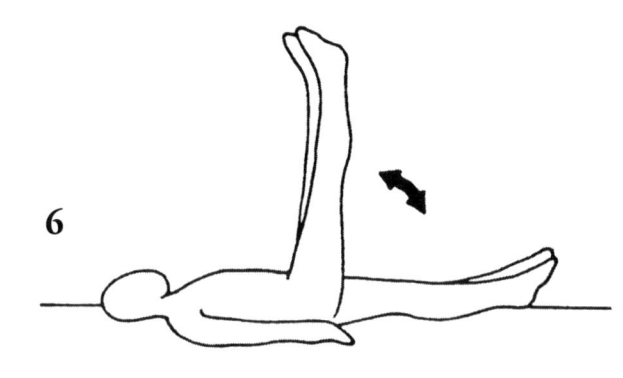

3

6

1. Lie down on the right side of your body. Raise the left leg up straight and catch it with both hands. Pull on the raised leg while keeping both legs straight. Inhale through the nose and exhale through the mouth heavily. Breathe loud and clear. 2 Minutes.

2. Lie down flat on your back and put your hands under your neck. Raise both legs to 6 inches and lower them rapidly with a heavy Breath of Fire. The legs will move up and down as quickly as the breath. Breath and legs move at the same time and rhythmically. "Breathe and move! . . . Create a music (as the feet hit the ground)." 6 Minutes. The yogis believe that this exercise will only hurt if your spleen is enlarged and that means that the spleen wants help.

3. Still lying on your back with the hands tightly clasped under your neck, begin sit-ups raising your torso up to 90 degrees and lowering it. Inhale as you rise up and exhale as you lie back down. "Coordinate the breath with the movement." Do 52 sit-ups. (Approximately 4 minutes.)

4. Remain on your back and relax. Breathe through your navel point and transport your energy through it. "Project slowly and react slowly. Bring a balance to the navel point." (Yogi Bhajan played the gong during this meditation.) 6 1/2 Minutes.

5. Remain on your back and chant in a monotone, using the power of the tip of the tongue: "Har, Har, Har, Har, Har, Har, Hari." (one repetition of the mantra takes about 3 seconds). 4 Minutes.

6. Stay on your back and immediately inhale and hold the breath while you slowly raise both legs to 90 degrees and lower them five times. (about 20 seconds) Inhale, hold the breath and slowly raise and lower both legs ten times. (about 25 seconds) Inhale, hold the breath and raise and lower the legs fifteen times. (about 30 seconds) Exhale and relax.

The inside organs need to be moved, not just your muscles. The inner organs must be stimulated... They must understand and reorganize their supplies.

Yogi Bhajan

Let the Liver Live

January 30, 1985

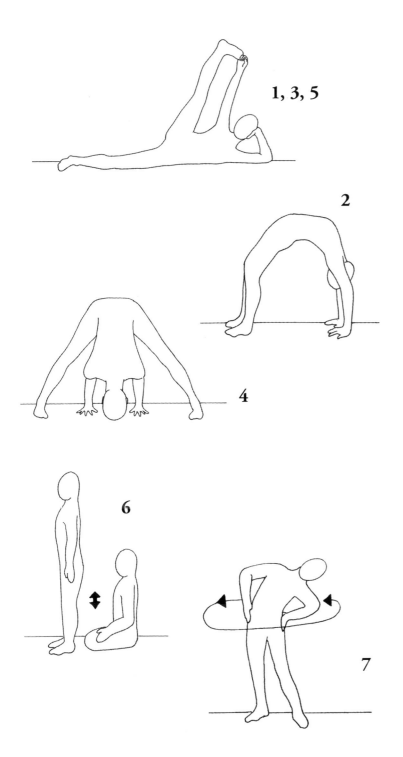

1, 3, 5

2

4

6

7

1. Lie on your left side and put your hand under your head. Lift your right leg up straight and hold your toe with your right hand, keeping both legs straight. Keep your left leg on the ground. Breath of Fire. 3 1/2 Minutes. "Relax the system so that the liver can change the boil and reorganize itself and connect with the spleen."

2. Half Wheel Pose. (Hands and feet flat on floor, body arched up.) Breathe in and out through the mouth, then in and out through the nose. Continue alternating from mouth to nose, taking one complete breath with each. 5 minutes.

3. Lie on your left side in the same position as exercise #1. Hold the position and do Breath of Fire through your mouth. 2 Minutes.

4. Stand up with your legs wide apart. Bend forward and stretch your hands back between your legs as far back as you can. Put your palms and your head on the ground and balance yourself. Hold this position for 1 Minute. Then, still in this position, roll your tongue, and do Breath of Fire through the rolled tongue. 3 1/2 Minutes.

5. Lie on your left side in the same position as exercise #1. Hold the position, make your mouth into a firm "O" shape and do a powerful and rapid Breath of Fire through the mouth (Cannon Breath). 1 Minute.

6. Stand up and sit down 52 times without using your hands for support. (1 count = 2 seconds)

7. Remain standing and place your hands on your hips. Roll your upper torso in large counter-clockwise circles. 2 Minutes.

Yogi Bhajan said, "Anybody who shall do exercise #7 for 11 minutes in the morning and 11 minutes at night will have no problem with Mr. Liver. Whosoever will do this set will be set for the rest of life."

Try to understand: when you do not consciously relate to your body, your mind consciously does not relate to you... When you do not control your mind consciously, your soul has no relationship with you. When your soul doesn't have a relationship with you, your actions can fall into the pit of depression, anger, and reaction. These are the three main things which bring pain into your life.

Yogi Bhajan

Toning The Kidneys

October 24, 1984

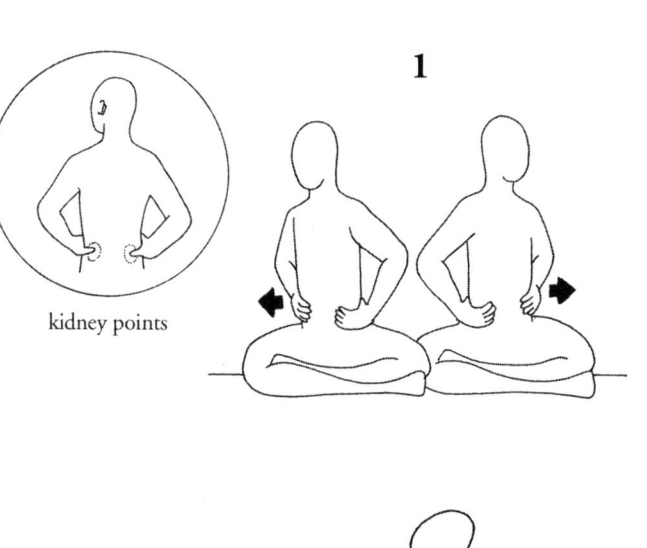

kidney points

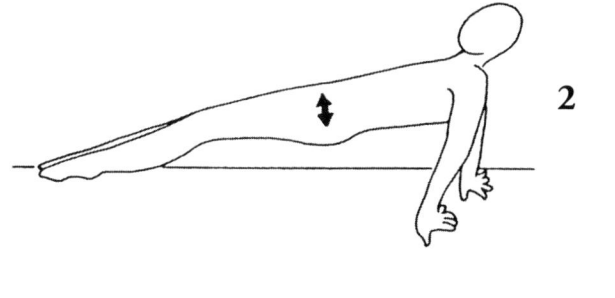

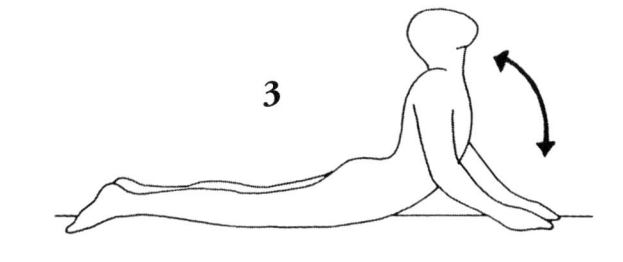

1. Sit in Easy Pose, hands grasping the waist, applying full pressure with your thumbs where your kidneys are. Twist left and right with a double breath. Inhale and exhale powerfully as you twist left and inhale and exhale powerfully as you twist right. This swing puts pressure at the kidneys and helps flush them out with each breath. Continue for 5 1/2 Minutes.

2. Immediately come into Back Platform Pose. Raise and lower your buttocks rapidly with Breath of Fire. Continue for 4 Minutes. This gives relief to the kidneys.

3. Immediately come into Cobra Pose. Then, in rhythm with Breath of Fire, raise yourself from flat on your stomach up into Cobra and lower yourself back down to flat on your stomach. Breathe heavily. Continue the movement for 2 Minutes.

4. Come into Easy Pose, mentally meditate on the sound of "Ek Ong Kaar." Concentrate at both the third eye point and the navel, and on the flow of energy up and down between these two points. 4 Minutes.

Then begin to chant as loud as you can: "Ek Ong Kaar Sat Gur Prasaad, Sat Gur Prasaad, Ek Ong Kaar" all in one breath. 2 Minutes.
(Yogi Bhajan played the gong throughout this entire meditation.)

To finish: inhale deeply, hold the breath for 15 seconds, and then keep the breath held another 10 seconds while you move the navel. Exhale and relax.

Those for whom God is the security, they shall always merge in God.

Yogi Bhajan

To Make the Skin Radiant

February 26, 1986

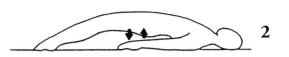

just knees

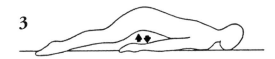

knees and arms

1

2

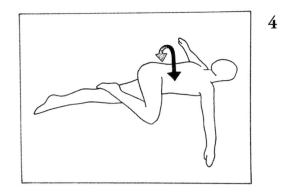

3

4

1. Sit with your legs stretched out in front of you, arms at your sides. Keeping the heels on the ground, bend the left knee and raise it. Then as you lower the left knee, raise the right knee so that you alternatively move the knees up and down very fast for 30 Seconds. Move directly into the next part of the exercise without stopping the leg motion.

Stretch the arms straight out in front of you, palms facing down and alternately move the hands and arms up and down coordinating with the leg motion. Move at a speed of 5 times per second or faster. "You have to bring the body to the point of sweating... It will open up the glandular system to a full capacity load, if you do it right." 5 Minutes.

2. Remain on your back and place your arms at your sides. Raise and lower your pelvis so that the buttocks are lifted off the ground and then dropped back down. Hammer the floor with your buttocks. Move very quickly. (2 count = 1 second) 2 Minutes.

3. Lie on your stomach with your arms at your sides. Raise and lower your pelvis so that the body, from hips to shoulders, jumps up and down rhythmically. 3 Minutes. Stimulate your circulation and make your cheeks "red like tomatoes".

4. Cat stretch alternately to the left side and then to the right side. Move quickly. Do as many as you can. 1 Minute.

5. Lie down with your arms by your sides and relax your whole body. "Breathe extremely slowly. Meditate and let your body go." 6 Minutes. Yogi Bhajan played the gong along with Singh Kaur's version of "Wahe Guroo, Wahe Guroo, Wahe Guroo, Wahe Jio."

To finish: roll your feet and hands and slowly get up.

Note: the times given above are the times for the exercises when the set was taught. Yogi Bhajan told the class that this set should be done proportionately for forty-five minutes. In this forty-five minute time period the first part of exercise #1 would be 2 Minutes. The second part of exercise #1 would be 18 Minutes. Exercise #2 would be 9 Minutes. Exercise #3 would be 12 Minutes. Exercise #4 would be 4 Minutes.

We are very much under stress, which is a part of our life. It is a state of mind which we definitely create between a reality and a non-reality...Lot of people are angry inside. People are not willing to admit the part they play in their own life for their own misery. I call it 'sophisticated misery.' We create it. We pay for it and we are part of it. Having realized that and seeing people go through that, I have realized how effectively it works on the skin and the metabolism...The main chakras that are affected by all this episode are the first, second, and third. They take the worst beating.

Yogi Bhajan

39

Owner's Manual

The Art of Equilibrium of the Stomach

May 8, 1985

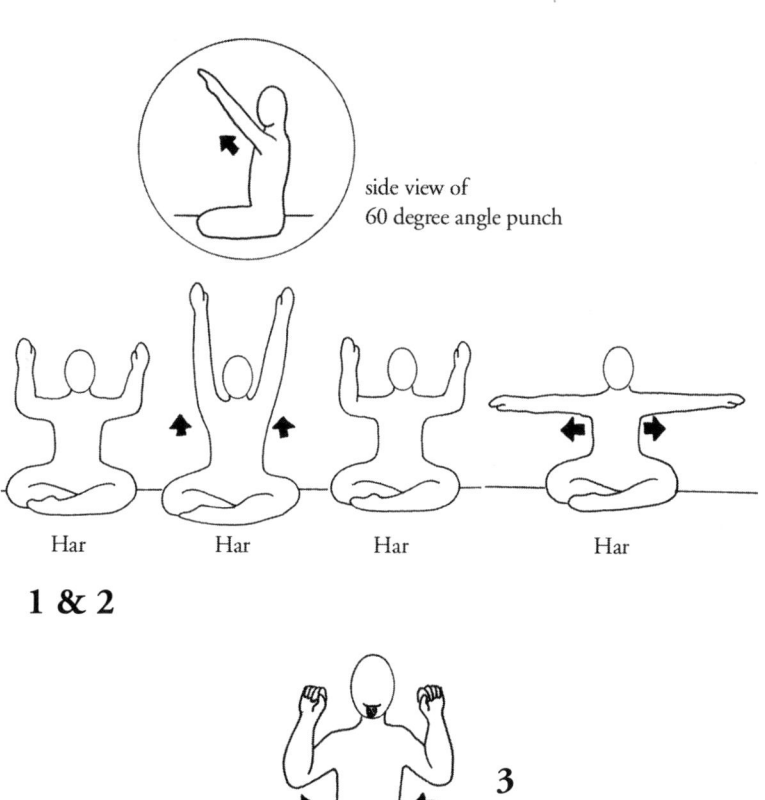

side view of
60 degree angle punch

Har   Har   Har   Har

1 & 2

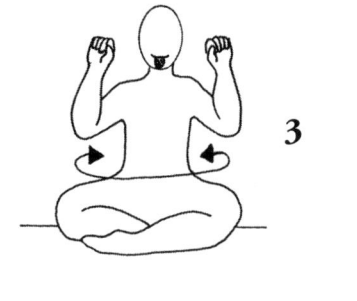

3

4

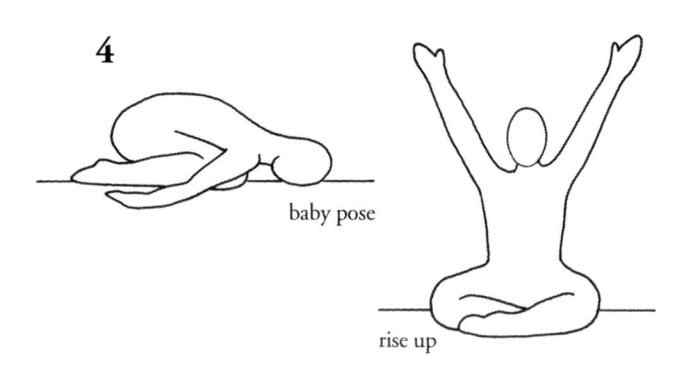

baby pose

rise up

1. Sitting in Easy Pose, bend the elbows bringing the hands shoulder width apart at the level of the ears. With a quick motion like a punch (but keeping both hands open), shoot the arms up and to the front at a 60 degree angle. Return the arms and hands to the first position and then repeat the punching motion out to the sides, parallel to the ground. Use outward force. These movements stretch the elbow, making it about two millimeters longer. After 1 Minute, begin to chant "Har" at each position using the tip of the tongue and the power of the navelpoint. Continue for 2 1/2 Minutes more. "Stomach is a fire. Get the anger out!"

2. Repeat Exercise 1, extending the tongue out of your mouth each time you chant "Har" at each position. (4 counts of "Har" = 2 seconds) Punch with anger and force. Get mad! 2 1/2 Minutes. (Yogi Bhajan demonstrated this way of chanting "Har" using a high pitch, like a falsetto.)

3. Bend the arms at a 90 degree angle at the elbow with the hands in fists held near the ears, twist the body left and right. Keep the tongue extended out of the mouth and chant "Har" with each twist. Go mad! 1 1/2 Minutes.

4. Get into Baby Pose with your forehead on the floor. Be relaxed and sleepy, while you chant "Har Har Mukande" from the navel for 9 1/2 Minutes. (Avtar Singh's version of the mantra was played in class.) Keep your tongue alive with the sound. (Yogi Bhajan played the gong.) Then rise up to Easy Pose, extend the arms up at approximately a sixty-degree angle to the sides and continue to chant. 1 1/2 Minutes. Inhale, hold your breath for 10 seconds, and exhale.

If you do not know the art of equilibrium of your stomach, you have not lived...The entire creative sensitivity of the body is in the stomach...It is the stomach that sends a message to the brain to coordinate the entire system...Rishi Taanaan found that the heart and brain are subject to the stomach... When the ancient yogis learned this fact, they developed a whole science of fasting and food combining... Because when you are emotional, you feel bad in stomach. When you are angry, you feel bad in stomach. This is agn granthi, this is where your life and fire is...The elbow area controls

5

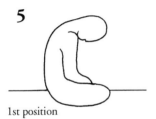

1st position

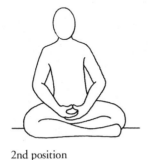

2nd position

5. Remaining in Easy Pose, put your hands in your lap and allow your head to hang totally relaxed, let your shoulders drop. Feel very tired and very sad. "Bring all the sadness out." Silently meditate on meditative music for 3 1/2 Minutes.

Stay in position and begin to chant with Kulwant Singh's version of "Chattr Chakkr Vartee" Healing Sounds of the Ancients, Volume I (see page 50). 3 Minutes.

Then sit up straight, feel exalted, magnify, sanctify, and glorify yourself and continue to chant for 3 more Minutes. (Yogi Bhajan played the gong, instructing the students to keep the mantra going, no matter how loud the gong became.)

To finish: Inhale, hold the breath for 30 seconds or longer and exhale. Repeat this breath sequence three more times.

Practicing this set regularly "will take away fear from your personality. Sadness and fear will fly away."

the stomach and this yoga set opens up the elbow to work on the stomach. (Yogi Bhajan indicated his upper arm from elbow to shoulder.)

Yogi Bhajan

Strengthening the Stomach

October 31, 1984

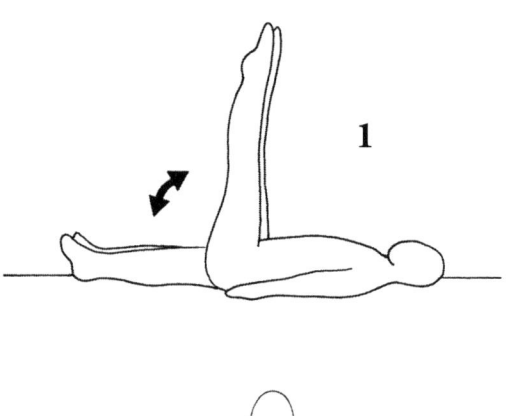

1. Lie on your back, heels together, lift both legs 90 degrees as you inhale through the mouth, then lower the legs as you exhale through the nose.
Continue for 3 1/2 Minutes (Keep your legs straight, with no bend in the knees).
Powerfully oxygenate your system. "This breath moves the pituitary in reverse order."

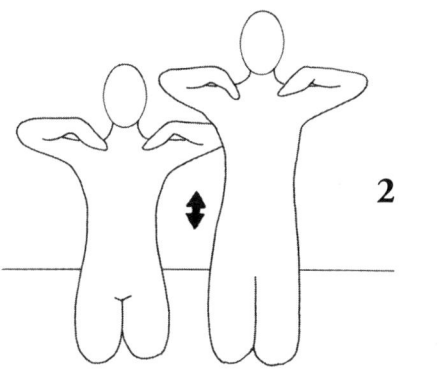

2. Sit on your heels in Rock Pose with your hands on your shoulders. Inhale through the mouth as you rise up to a kneeling position, exhale through the nose as you return to Rock Pose. Continue for 3 1/2 Minutes. Move quickly and powerfully. Bring some relaxation "to the back side of your knees where all tension is just a problem."

3. Sit in Easy Pose with your hands on your knees. Grind your stomach around in wide counter-clockwise circles, moving powerfully. Move the lower back. Lose weight! Lose fat! Clean your digestive system. Move! Continue for 4 Minutes.

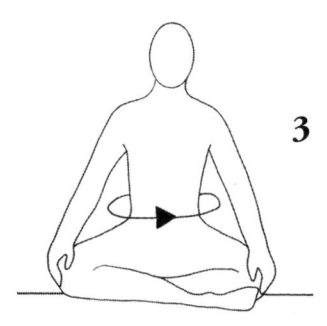

4. Remain in Easy Pose and interlock your hands behind your back. Inhale through the mouth as you bend forward into Yoga Mudra, bringing your forehead to the ground in front of you and raising your arms up. Exhale through the nose as you come back into Easy Pose and lower your arms. Continue for 3 1/2 Minutes. "It will create the balance of the imbalanced energy." Move quickly.

5. Lie flat on your back. Meditatively project at the navel point. Vibrate the energy there. (Yogi Bhajan played the gong for this meditation). 8 1/2 Minutes.

6. Wake yourself up. Roll your hands around your wrists and your feet around your ankles briefly. Bring your knees to your chest and briefly roll on your spine. Bring your knees to your chest and then extend the legs out, stretching the legs forward and back a few times.

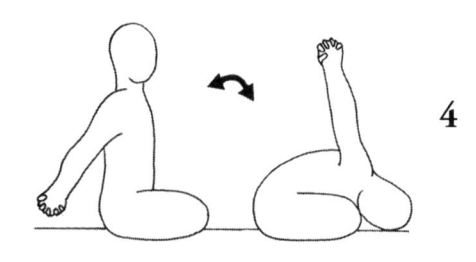

Stomach is a very powerful organ in the body... The stomach secretes juices. The idea is that for the first eighteen years, those juices are very heavy. So metabolism is very perfect. Whatever you eat, you can digest. There is never a problem. The second eighteen years, you somehow digest what you eat. You understand that, so you eat and drink and wine and dine, and you consider yourself super-right. After that you start paying the cost. Your metabolism starts changing and your digestive system starts changing. Your liver cannot do the work. Food cannot be digested and eliminated within twenty-four hours. You think you are only responsible for eating... You don't think you are responsible for eliminating. Anything that remains within your body for more than twenty-four hours will poison your body. That is the main cause of all your problems.

Yogi Bhajan

Build up the Glandular System and Inner Organs

November 21, 1984

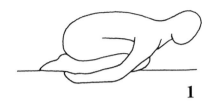

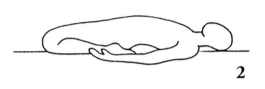

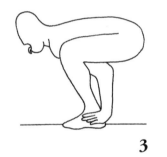

1. Baby Pose: Sit on your heels, with your forehead on the ground and your arms resting at your sides pointing backward. Lift up your neck and do a strong Breath of Fire from the navel point. 3 Minutes. "Breath of Fire has to be real from the navel point. It is difficult."

2. From Baby Pose, lean back until you are lying on your back (but still with your heels underneath your buttocks) and do Breath of Fire. 3 Minutes. "If you cannot do this, you are old, irrespective of your age. And whether you like me or not, keep this posture alive because this is the secret posture in which body metabolism will not be in a position to kill you."

3. Chair Pose. With your feet shoulder width apart and flat on the ground, squat down so the your back is parallel to the floor. Reach back between your thighs and grasp your heels with your fingertips pointing forward. In this position, stick your tongue way out and do Breath of Fire through the mouth. 3 Minutes.

During the Har meditation Yogi Bhajan played the gong and he said,"The inner vibration of the sound of the gong is that mantra, is the heart center."

"Make this set a part of your life for eleven minutes every day. (Eleven minutes means three minutes for each exercise and two minutes for transitioning from exercise to exercise.) You will never have problems with a lot of your main organs. Glands are the guardians of the health. These three postures are essentially required by every human being up to the age of ninety-five...This set will make your mind fresh. It will take away your fear. You will have `grit.' You will experience yourself...Do it anytime, but you must do it. If you cannot do it, perfect it. Slowly and gradually the body will adapt to it. It means the body has the capacity to heal itself. Mind has the capacity to heal itself."

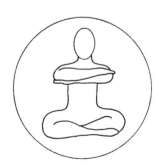

NOTE: You can extend this set into a full class, by keeping the time for each exercise to 3 minutes, and then adding a five minute relaxation. Repeat the sequence twice more, making a total of three repetitions. For the final five minute relaxation, sit in Easy Pose with your arms at shoulder height parallel to the ground, palms down, right arm resting on left while you breathe very, very slowly. Concentrate at the third eye point. Silently, mentally, chant "Haree" 84 times on the inhalation, and silently mentally chant "Har" 84 times on the exhalation. (The inhale and exhale are about 10-15 seconds each.) "Haree" calls upon the creative energy and "Har" is joining the God within and without.

What happens is, according to age, the cells of the body stop regenerating themselves within the time limit that the metabolism wants. First indication is your metabolism is not functioning as it should be. Second indication is that your body starts depositing fat below your navel point, that means that your liver is not as active as it should be. Third is that your weight starts increasing. And after that one organ or the other will be in question. And you think it is normal. That is the worst.

Yogi Bhajan

To Build Stamina and Spark the Glandular System

KWTC July 15, 1985

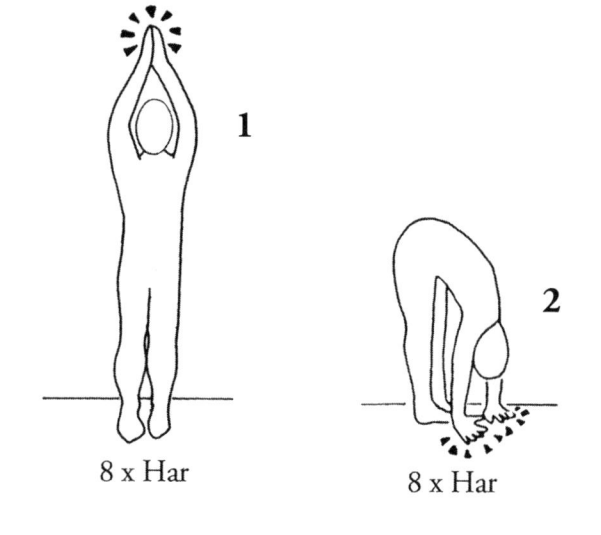

1 — 8 x Har

2 — 8 x Har

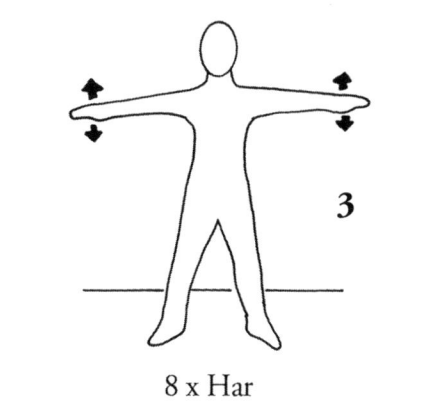

3 — 8 x Har

1. Standing with feet together, clap your hands over your head 8 times (about 4 seconds). Each time you clap, chant "Har" with the tip of your tongue.

2. Bend over and beat the ground with both hands hard, 8 times(about 4 seconds). With each pat, chant "Har" with the tip of your tongue. "Get high on it!"

3. Stand up straight up with arms out to the sides parallel to the ground. Raise and lower the arms a few inches, patting the air with a strong pressure. Chant "Har" with the tip of the tongue 8 times. (One complete up and down movement is one "Har" and 8 repetitions of "Har" take about 4 seconds)

4. Criss-cross the arms and legs chanting "Har", both as the arms and legs cross and when they are out at the sides for a total of 8 chants of "Har."(about 4 seconds) Move the arms and legs fully.

These first four exercises can be practiced as a set all by themselves. To do so, move directly through all four exercises and then start again at the beginning. Continue cycling through all the exercises for 11-31 Minutes.

"This set will give you rest. The clapping is for the brain, it is the best massage of the meridians. It will benefit your colon, stomach, spleen, and liver. It is very essential that you do it."

Purpose of life is to remain harmonious against the most unharmonious challenge. Happiness is an in-between process. Happiness you cannot 'get'. If you develop yourself to remain harmonious against the most unharmonious environment, happy you are automatically. There is no problem.

Yogi Bhajan

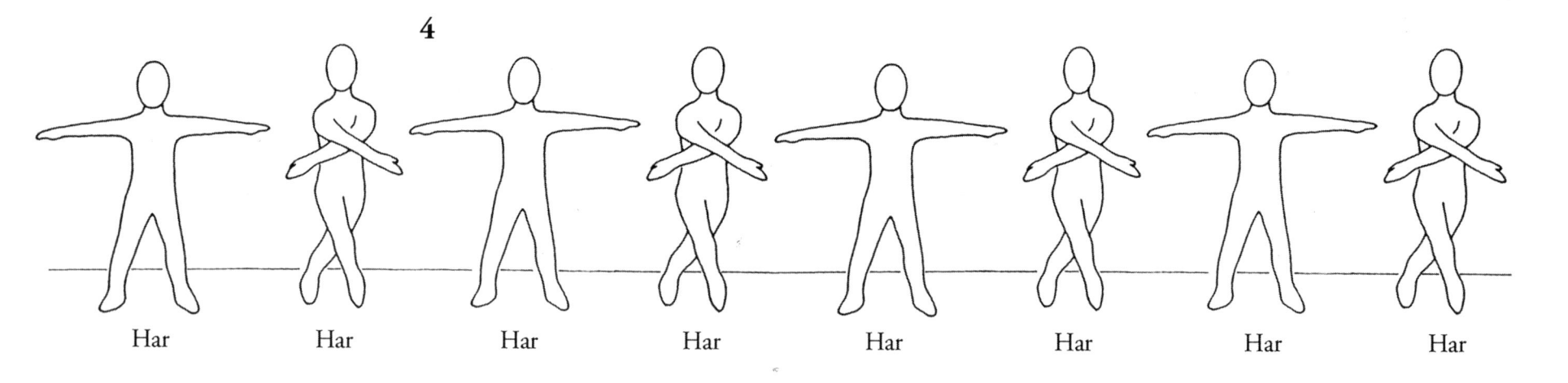

4

Har   Har   Har   Har   Har   Har   Har   Har

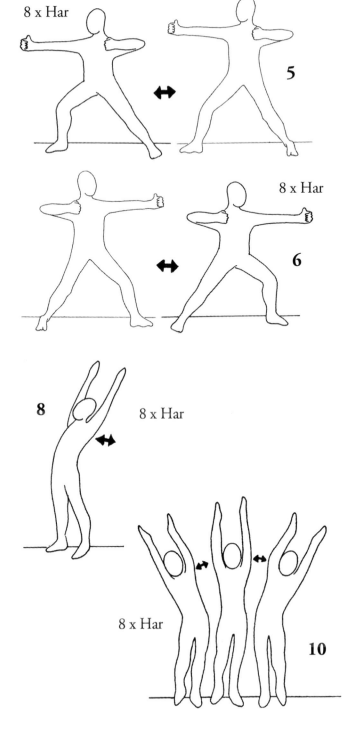

The following section was taught on July 16th and it was combined with the first four exercises taught on July 15th to work out the whole body. Yogi Bhajan called it the "elementary woman exercise." It stimulates the 12 glands and builds stamina. When it was first taught at KWTC 1985, the women practiced the complete set for one hour each day. This second series of exercises is good for the colon, the metabolism, and the lymph glands. Yogi Bhajan said that in five or six rounds of this combined exercise set, the whole body will be done, but a person should be able to do this for a total of 62 Minutes with a break after 31 Minutes.

5. Do Archer Pose with the right leg forward. Bend the right knee, extending in and out of the full stretch of the position, chanting "Har" with the tip of the tongue 8 times (about 6 seconds).

6. Repeat Archer Pose with the left knee forward, chanting "Har" with the tip of the tongue 8 times (about 6 seconds).

7. Repeat exercise # 4

8. With the arms in the air over the head, bend backwards 8 times chanting "Har." (about 6 seconds).

9. Repeat exercise # 4

10. With the arms straight up over the head, bend to the right 4 times chanting "Har" each time and then bend to the left 4 times chanting "Har" each time, keeping the arms somewhat close to the head. (8-10 seconds)

11. Relax on the back with your knees to your chest, locking your legs with your hands and go to sleep. As you relax, listen to a recording of "Dhan Dhan Ram Das Gur."

On July 17th Yogi Bhajan gave the particular layout listed above after the sixty-two minute version of this combined set and he called it "Vayu Praan Nidra". "It is very rare, but for every female, it is essential. You must go in this once in a while." This layout was done listening to a recording of "Dhan Dhan Ram Das Gur" and lasted forty-five minutes.

There are twelve glands in you. Those glands are the guardians of your health (mind, body, and soul, whatever you want to call it), because... they secrete with the blood and make the combination. If you cannot stimulate these twelve glands one day or another, you can be caught by disease or weakness.

Normally as a woman you don't put pressure on the thighs. That's your greatest weakness. The thigh bone controls the calcium, magnesium, sodium, and potassium... These four major elements are responsible for making you a woman.

Yogi Bhajan

45

Owner's Manual

Glandular System Tune-up

August 21, 1985

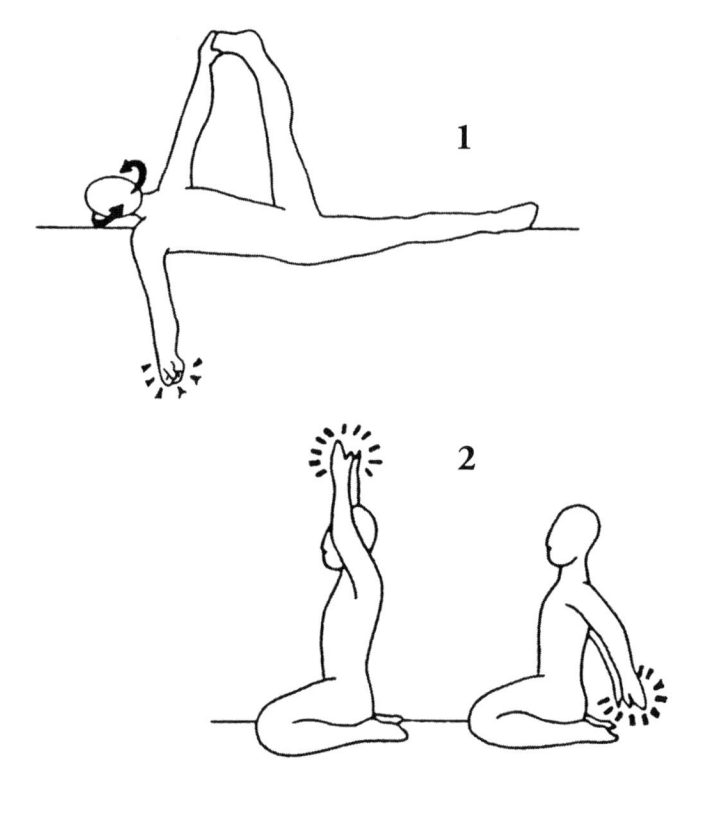

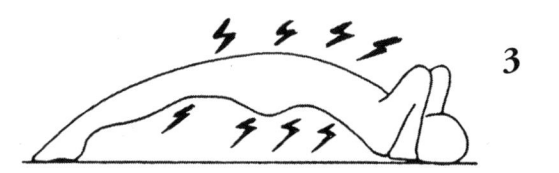

1. Lie down on your right side. Lift your left leg straight up and grab the toes of your left foot with your left hand. Now stretch your right arm straight out from your body and make a fist. Begin simultaneously rolling your neck and clenching and opening your fist. "Hand has to be a pumping machine." Pump blood to your neck, work your thyroid. 2 1/2 Minutes.

2. Sit on your heels, reach behind and clap your hands together at the small of your back and then raise your arms and clap your hands over your head. Chant SA TA NA MA, chant a syllable with each clap. (one complete SA-TA-NA-MA = 2 seconds) "Stretch the sciatica at the shoulder points." 3 1/2 Minutes.

3. Meen Mudra (fish exercise) : lie down on your back, clasping your hands under your neck and begin jumping your body around like a jumping fish, move any and every part of your body vigorously so that you can "let the system relax, let the glands work it out." 2 1/2 Minutes.

4. Sitting in Easy Pose with hands clasped, raise both arms up in front of you. Using your arms like a hammer, raise them up over your head and forcefully hit them toward the ground (without actually hitting the ground) and then raise them up again over your head. Continue moving forcefully. "Get angry and get going!...Get mad. Take the anger out." 4 Minutes.

The more forceful your grip and the more powerful and controlled your hammer blow, the better the effect on your heart. "It is the relationship between the heart and the sciatica."

We want you to live the light of your life in reality. Therefore you have to change your attitudes. With the modern trend, with the heavy pressures, sex is not the way. You have to transform sexual energy into the sixth sense of your own exalted common sense. You have to understand that there is only "x" amount of energy which you can use for all the purposes of your life. You cannot drag it down. You have to purposefully look at yourself and make yourself important to you, around you, and for you. Let this be the day and let this be the beginning of that goal to achieve.

Yogi Bhajan

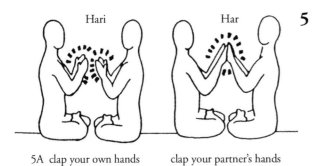

Hari   Har   **5**

5A clap your own hands   clap your partner's hands

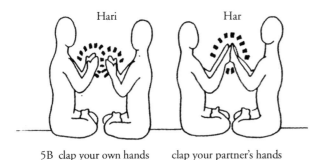

Hari   Har

5B clap your own hands   clap your partner's hands

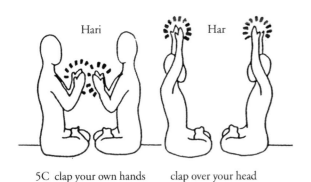

Hari   Har

5C clap your own hands   clap over your head

5. Exercise for the brain: get a partner and sit facing each other

A. Clap your hands together in front of your chest and then clap your partners hands (like patty cake.)

B. Clap your own hands again and clap your partner's hands.

C. Clap your own hands again and then raise your own arms up and clap your own hands together over your head. And continue this sequence. 3 Minutes.

Then continue the motion chanting "Hari Har" once as you perform A chanting "Hari Har" once as you perform B and again chanting "Hari Har" once as you perform C. 2 1/2 Minutes. (One repetition of "Hari Har" = 3 seconds.) Chant from the navel.

During exercise number five, Yogi Bhajan said,"This is how they used to teach us mantras. Actually it is a brain exercise. It is the exercise which makes the gray matter and the serum in the spine to combine in circulation and it is a very good thing."

6. Sit on your heels and interlock your fingers in front of your chest, palms down, and shake every part of your body. Close your eyes and go wild. 3 Minutes. "Give your nervous system a renewed strength...Shake your body like it has never been shaken."

Continued next page

6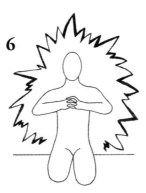

47

Owner's Manual

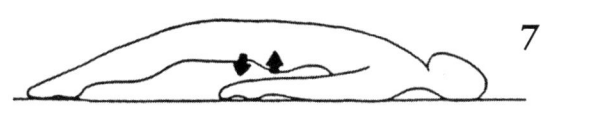

7

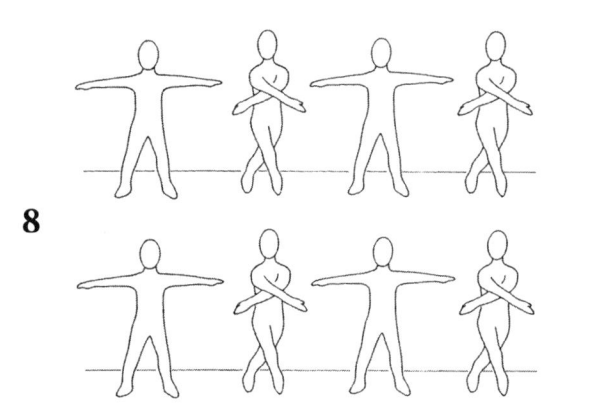

8

Repeat pages 44-45

10

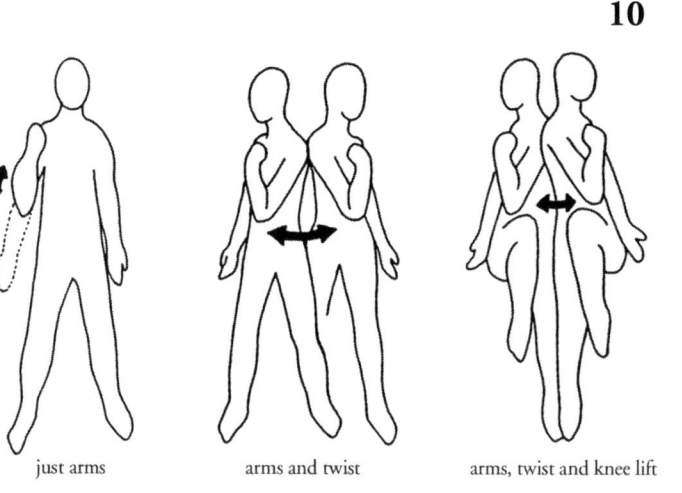

just arms   arms and twist   arms, twist and knee lift

7. Lie down on your back and quickly bounce your hips up and down on the floor. 1 1/2 Minutes. "Twist it. Dance it. Left and right. Right and left."

8. Move quickly through exercise #1-10 of the yoga set called "To Build Stamina and Spark the Glandular System" (see pages 44-45) Cycle through this sequence for 5 1/2 Minutes.

9. Relax for 4 Minutes.

10. Stand in front of a mirror. Have your arms at your sides with the palms of your hands facing forward. Make a fist of your right hand and bend your elbow, bringing your fist to your shoulder. Lower your right hand and relax the fist while you make a fist of your left hand and bring it to your shoulder. Continuing this movement, twist your torso from the waist: twisting to the left when your right fist comes up and twisting to the right when your left fist comes up. Once those two movements are coordinated, begin lifting the left knee up as you twist to the left and bring the right fist up. As you twist to the right, bring the right knee up as the left fist comes up. This is to be aerobic movement so move quickly. 3 Minutes.

11. Long Deep Relaxation in Corpse Pose, lying down flat on your back. Make your breath long and go to sleep. 7 Minutes.

Yogi Bhajan played the gong for the first two and a half minutes of this layout, then he instructed the class to nap at their own command for the last four and a half minutes. "Learning to nap yourself for three minutes is one of the greatest relaxations you can give to your system."

Music & Mantras

If you do not have the specific version of the music played in a set, you may substitute other meditative Kundalini Yoga music or do the set without music. To hear the correct pronunciation of an individual mantra used in this manual, please visit www.kriteachings.org and click on "Tools for Students and Teachers" and then on "Aquarian Teacher Mantra Pronunciation."

Dhan Dhan Ram Das Gur

Dhan dhan Raam Daas Gur, jin siria tineh savaariaa
Poore hoee karamaat, aap sireejana-haaray dhaariaa
Sikhee ateh sangatee, paarabrahm kar namaskaariaa
Atal ataao atol too, tayraa ant na paaravaariaa
Jinee too sayviaa bhao kar, say tudh paar utaaria
Labh lobh kaam krodh moho, maar kadhe tudh sapaaravaariaa
Dhan so tayraa taan heh, sach tayraa pehsakaariaa
Nanak too(n) Lehenaa too(n) heh, Gur Amar too(n) veecharria
Guru ditta taa man saadhaariaa

Blessed, blessed is Guru Ram Das
The Lord who created Thee, He alone has adorned Thee
Complete is Thy miracle.
The Creator Himself has installed Thee on the throne.
Deeming Thee as the Transcendent Lord, Thine followers and congregations bow before Thee.
Thou are immovable, unfathomable, and immeasurable.
Thou hast no end or bounds.
They who serve Thee with love,
Them Thou ferriest across.
Avarice, covetousness, sexual desire, wrath and wordly love,
Thou hast beaten and driven out with all their ramifications.
Praiseworthy is Thy place
True are Thine bounties.
Thou are Nanak, Thou art Angad
Thou art Guru Amar Das, so do I deem thee.
When I saw the Guru, then was my soul sustained.

Ek Ong Kaar Sat Gur Prasaad, Sat Gur Prasaad, Ek Ong Kaar
The Creator and the Creation are One.
This is experienced through the True Guru's Grace.

Ek Ong Kaar Sat Naam, Siri Wahe Guroo
There is one Creator, Truth is His Name, great is His wisdom.

Guroo, Guroo, Wahe Guroo, Guru Ram Das Guroo
Great is Guru Ram Das

Har
The power of God

Har, Har, Har, Har, Har, Haray
God, God, God, God, Who manifested the Creation

Har Har Mukande
God the liberator

Haree
God in Creative Action

Har Har Gobinde, Har Har Mukande
Har Har Udare, Har Har Apaare
Har Har Hariang, Har Har Kariang
Har Har Nirnaame, Har Har Akaame

God the Sustainer, God the Liberator
God the Enlightener, God the Infinite
God the Destroyer, God the Creator
God the Nameless, God the Desireless

Jaap Sahib
A musical prayer of the Sikhs.

Jai Te Gan

Khag khand bihandan, khal dal khandar at ran mandan bar bandan.
Bhujadand akhandan, tayj prachandan jot amandan, bhaan prabhan.
Sukh santaa karnan, durmat darnan kilabikh harnan, as sarnan.
Jai jai jag kaaran, srisht ubaaran nam pratipaaran jai tay gan.

You conquer countries and destroy wicked armies.
You are the beautiful adornment of the righteous soldier.
Your arm is unstoppable. Your brightness resplendent.
Your radiance and splendor rival the sun.
You bestow peace among saints and terrify the wicked.
You dispell evil and are my hope and protection.
Hail the Creator of the Universe, liberator of all Creation.
You are my protector, hail the holy sword of God.

Last Four Lines of Jaap Sahib

Chattr chakkr vartee, chattr chakkr bhugatay
Suyambhav subhang, sarab daa sarab jugatay,
Dukaalang pranaasee, dayaalang saroopay,
Sada ang sangay, abhangang bibhootay

Thou art pervading in all the four quarters of the Universe,
Thou art the Enjoyer in all the four quarters of the Universe,
Thou art Self-illumined and united with all,
Destroyer of bad times, embodiment of mercy, Thou art ever within us.
Thou art the everlasting Giver of indestructible power.

Mool Mantra

Ek Ong Kaar, Sat Naam, Kartaa Purakh, Nirbho, Nirvair, Akaal Moort, Ajoonee Saibhang, Gurprasaad. Jap. Aad such, jugaad such, haibhee such, Nanaak hosee bhee such.

The Creator and all the Creation are One. This is our true identity. God is the doer of all. Beyond fear, beyond revenge. Of undying form, unborn, self –illumined, complete in the Self. This is realized by Guru's Grace. Repeat the Naad. True in the beginning. True throughout the ages. True at this moment. Nanak says that this shall ever be true.

Rakhay Rakhanahaar

Rakhay rakhanahaar aap ubaarian, Guru ke pairee paa-ay kaaj savaarian Hoa aap dayaal manaho naa(n) visaari-an, saad janaa kai , sang bhavjal taarian, Saakat nindak dusht khin maaeh bidaarian, tis sahib kee tayk Nanak manai maaeh Jis simrat sukh hoay sagalay dookh jaaeh.

Oh, God, You save us all and take us across, uplifting and giving excellence. You gave us the touch of the Lotus Feet of the Guru, and all our jobs are done with perfection. You have become merciful, kind, and compassionate; and so our mind does not forget You. In the company of the holy, you take us from misfortune and calamities, scandal and disrepute. That great Lord is my anchor. Nanak, keep Him firmly in my mind. By meditating and repeating His Name, all happiness comes and all sorrows and pain go away.

Sa Ta Na Ma
Infinity, birth, death, rebirth

Sat Naam
Truth is God's Name

Wahe Guroo , Wahe Guroo , Wahe Guroo , Wahe Jio
The experience of the Divine Wisdom is ecstasy. My soul is in ecstasy.

Music can be purchased from your local yoga center or the following mail order companies:

Spirit Voyage
www.spiritvoyage.com
888-735-4800

Ancient Healing Ways
www.a-healing.com
800-359-2940

Resources

The Kundalini Research Institute: Your Source for
Kundalini Yoga as Taught by Yogi Bhajan®
Teacher Training, Online Resources, Publishing, and Research

www.kundaliniresearchinstitute.org

The Yogi Bhajan Library of Teachings
Keeping the Legacy Alive! Donate Today!

www.kundaliniresearchinstitute.org

For information regarding international events:

www.3HO.org

To find a teacher in your area or for more information
about becoming a Kundalini Yoga teacher:

www.kundaliniyoga.com

Of further interest:

www.sikhnet.org

Kundalini Yoga as taught by Yogi Bhajan®

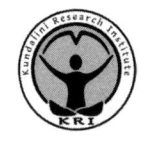

Kundalini Research Institute